MW01122336

Assessment in Residential Care for Children and Youth

Residential treatment for children and youth (RTCY) programs not only need to be explored for the efficacy of the programs, but also in the actual assessment of various aspects of those programs. *Assessment in Residential Care for Children and Youth* provides practical information on the placement of children in residential care programs, the efficacy of those programs, staff issues, and outcomes for youths in the programs. Respected authorities examine issues on assessment upon entering residential care, treatment issues during care, and programmatic concerns from a larger systems perspective.

Unlike other resources on this topic, this book uniquely focuses solely on assessment. The book comprehensively offers strategies and practical assessment tools addressing the full spectrum of issues from the child's or youth's entrance in residential care to their exit, such as placement, treatment, and outcomes. This valuable text is extensively referenced and includes helpful figures and tables to clearly present data.

This book is a valuable resource for residential administrators, program directors and coordinators, counselors, and staff who have a role in assessing residential treatment programs for children and youth at any level.

This book was published as a special issue of *Residential Treatment for Children and Youth*.

Dr Roy Rodenhiser is Director of the School of Social Work at Boise State University, Idaho, USA.

Assessment in Residential Care for Children and Youth

Edited by Roy Rodenhiser

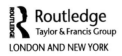

Routledge
Taylor & Francis Group
LONDON AND NEW YORK

First published 2009 by Routledge
2 Park Square, Milton Park, Abingdon, Oxon, OX14 4RN

Simultaneously published in the USA and Canada
by Routledge
270 Madison Avenue, New York, NY 10016

*Routledge is an imprint of the Taylor & Francis Group, an informa
business*

© 2009 Edited by Roy Rodenhiser

Typeset in Times by Value Chain, India
Printed and bound in the United States of America on acid-free paper
by IBT Global

British Library Cataloguing in Publication Data
A catalogue record for this book is available from the British Library

ISBN 10: 0-7890-3838-2 (h/b)
ISBN 10: 0-7890-3839-0 (p/b)
ISBN 13: 978-0-7890-3838-8 (h/b)
ISBN 13: 978-0-7890-3839-5 (p/b)

Assessment in Residential Care for Children and Youth

CONTENTS

Preface

When I made the proposal to be the editor of this volume, I had in mind a collection that provided the reader with quality assessment information that Residential Treatment for Children and Youth (RTCY) professionals might use in a practical way. I envisioned assessment chapters that provided the reader with useful information related to the placement of children, the efficacy of residential programs, staff issues in residential programs, and outcomes for youths in residential programs.

In waiting for prospective articles to arrive and with the help of my great administrative assistant Jessica Lantz I did a brief literature search of about 400 articles using the key words assessment, residential care, youth, children, and others. I found that of the 402 articles reviewed 202 explored the efficacy of treatment in residential programs. Only 22 articles explored assessing youth for placement and fewer yet, 17 explored youth after leaving their residential care facility. While the primary focus of the reviewed literature justifiably focuses on the efficacy of treatment, there seems a need for evaluation of how youth enter and exit the residential system. I also found substantive bodies of work that focused on the assessment of treatment for women with dependent children, and the majority of treatment programs found in this search were substance abuse treatment facilities. While this could be the start of another article by this writer, the review of the literature seems to indicate a need for more assessment in how youth enter the residential care system and how they fare after exit. It would be presumptuous of me to draw any conclusions until a thorough review of the literature is completed. My opinion now is there is a need for more assessment of RTCY programs at many levels: programmatic, staff, entrance, during treatment, and at exit.

The selected chapters for this collection typify what was found in the literature. Two examine issues related to assessment upon entering residential care, three examine treatment issues during care, and five examine programmatic concerns from a larger systems perspective.

James L. Wolk et al. start the assessment off with a look at the fidelity of the assessment processes and tools that were utilized across multiple sites to enhance therapeutic childcare interventions.

Two chapters with strength-based assessment strategies are presented by Rebecca G. Block and John D. Matthews who discuss the unique needs of GBL youth in residential care settings and William Barton et al. who describe a strengths-based assessment tool developed specifically for use in juvenile justice programs. Both of these have some elements of initial assessment (entrance) and treatment focus.

Two chapters discuss staff issues. Amy Levin and James T. Decker look at the rate of staff satisfaction as compared to client satisfaction in a residential treatment facility and Kristin Hurley et al. describe the development of the Staff Implementation Observation Form, an instrument to assess staff competence delivering an intervention to youth in group home care with behavioral or emotional disorders.

The remaining five chapters examine programmatic issues in RTCY. Stephen Wong discusses his assessment of official state program reviews for the types of behavior management and behavioral interventions being used and the extent to which agency practices were consistent with learning theory principles and you will find his results interesting. Loring Jones examines differences in two residential care giving models (houseparent vs. child care worker) in providing continuity of care for youth in residential placement, and the effect that a care giving model had on selected program outcomes. Timothy F. Page et al. describe a unique standardized clinical assessment using the point of view of children. It was developed to assess children's perceptions of their caregiving environments and it is called the Narrative Story-Stem Technique (NSST). JedMetzger describes the assessment and the process that led to the redesign of services at an upstate New York residential center and how evidence-based models were selected and integrated. W. Guy Tidwell discusses the application of functional behavioral assessment (FBA) to treatment of problem behavior in residential facilities.

I hope you enjoy the book and find it useful in your work. I would like to hear from our readers about future assessment plans and maybe even the need for a follow-up assessment volume. For all the dedicated professionals in RTCY, this collection only touches on the need for assessment in your profession and that in my editorial comments above I do not pretend to be speaking for the profession. I have the greatest respect for all of you working in RTCY.

Roy W. Rodenhiser, MSW, EdD
School of Social Work
Boise State University

Supporting the Fidelity of Assessment Tools in a Statewide Multisite Residential Substance Abuse Experience for Mothers and Their Children

James L. Wolk, DSW
Mary McLaughlin, LCSW
Sarah Dailey, LCSW

BACKGROUND

In 1996, the Personal Responsibility and Work Opportunities Reconciliation Act (PRWORA) was signed into law in order to "end welfare as we know it." Welfare programs nationally were redefined from entitlement programs to temporary assistance programs with an emphasis on returning policy responsibilities to state government and individuals to the workforce. In Georgia, the Temporary Assistance to Needy Families (TANF) program created a stringent 48-month lifetime limit for cash benefits. This added a greater sense of urgency to have mothers equipped to enter the workforce.

Accordingly, Georgia created a comprehensive collaborative in response to changes in income maintenance. The Department of Human Resources (DHR), the Department of Labor (DOL), and the Department of Technical and Adult Education (DTAE) joined forces to create a "job ready workforce." In addition to these three state agencies, the state submitted a plan to the United States Department of Labor to move longterm recipients of public assistance into jobs. This plan defined longterm recipients as: a recipient of TANF benefits for 30 or more months or would reach the 48-month lifetime maximum within 12 months and at least two of the following barriers–has not completed high school or a GED, low math or reading skills, poor work history, requires substance abuse treatment.

In partial response to this plan, the state of Georgia through an existing state collaboration of substance abuse treatment centers, created the Ready for Work (RFW) Substance Abuse Treatment Program. By removing substance abuse as a barrier to employment, and adding additional gender-specific services such as allowing children to accompany their mothers to treatment, it was believed this population would be better able to return to the workforce. One major component of this Ready for Work initiative was the development of 20 residential substance abusetreatment programs across Georgia for women and their children. These RFW Residential Substance Abuse Programs were located in urban, suburban, and rural areas of the state. They provided for a length of stay from 6-12 months and provided the following services: primary health care for the women and primary pediatric care for the children, gender specific substance abuse treatment for women which included issues of relationships, sexual and physical abuse, and parenting skills, employment readiness skills, case management and transportation, and therapeutic child care for children.

The need for specialized services for the children of substance abusing mothers is well documented (Metsch, 1995). In addition, there is a substantial amount of research indicating increased program completion and better client outcomes for mothers when their children are a part of the treatment process (Knight, Logan, & Simpson, 2001; Uziel-Miller, 2000; Connors, Bradley, & Whiteside-Mansell, 2001; Grella, Joslin, Hsu, 2000; Taylor & Francis, 2004; Scott-Lennox, Rose, Bohlig, & Lennox, 2000; Jackson, 1995). While there is some research in the literature on the usefulness of therapeutic childcare (Moore, Amsden, & Gogerty, 1998; Casey Foundation, 2001) the research on effective provision of this service is scarce.

Specifically, in an article by H. Westley Clark (2001), the director of the Center for Substance Abuse Treatment, Substance Abuse and Mental Health Services Administration (CSAT/SAMHSA) presents preliminary data collected in a national cross-site evaluation of 24 residential treatment programs for pregnant and postpartum women and their children. The evaluation found that the substance abuse, criminal activity and increased employment outcomes were positive at six months follow-up. The importance of residential treatment programs for women and children is evident and implications for future research include; using comparison groups to determine whether residential treatment and/or the specific treatments provided through the treatment programs are the most effective methods for treating this population and research focusing on the children of substance abusing women. Among other recommendations, Clark suggested that the future work of programs already in existence should include strengthening collaboration that benefit the children while in treatment with their mothers, developing experts who can provide appropriate care for the children of substance abusing mother, and developing appropriate screening and assessment instruments for early identification of problems in children.

It is in the above context that this paper will describe Georgia's multisite gender specific, residential substance abuse treatment program for women on TANF and their children. Specifically, this paper will focus on the programmatic and assessment challenges to the process of including children in the residential treatment of their mothers. The intent is to describe a process for designing an assessment protocol for children in this setting, but also describe the constraints on the collection and utility of a quality assessment tool for children in a multisite, somewhat unstable, adult-focused service delivery environment.

THERAPEUTIC CHILDCARE METHODOLOGY

As noted above, Georgia established the twenty, 6-12 month, gender specific, residential treatment programs for women and their children subsequent to the passage of welfare reform to remove the barriers to work. In addition to the clinical and support services to confront the mother's substance abuse problems and the vocational skills development, the programs were required to institute a therapeutic childcare program for the children in residence.

While there is no generally agreed upon definition of therapeutic childcare, the description offered by Child Care and Early Education Research Connection captures the intent of therapeutic childcare. It states that TCC is "child care services provided for at-risk children, such as children in homeless families, and in families with issues related to alcohol and substance abuse, violence, and neglect." They further note that therapeutic childcare is an integrated array of structured professional interventions conducted in a safe, nurturing, stimulating environment.

In order to increase understanding of issues confronting children in this therapeutic environment, a pilot study was initiated at 6 of the 20 sites. Six sites were selected based upon their geographic area, size of program and presence of clinical staff. Two of the sites selected were Metro Atlanta programs, two were small town programs, and two were rural programs. The involvement at these sites was aimed at increasing child *centered* services at each site. The therapeutic childcare consultations, conducted by a licensed clinical social worker, generally included chart reviews, assessment of services, clinical screening, group facilitation, and staff training in the use of assessment and or screening tools. Visits varied at the programs from once a week for a full day at half the sites to once a month for a half day at the other sites.

After a review of available screening instruments for children, the Denver II Developmental Screening tool was chosen. The choice of the Denver II was made based on a series of factors, the most compelling being that due to the lack of clinical staff on site the tool had to be easily used by trained para-professionals. The TCC Consultant's clinical knowledge of the test, ease of training users, and the ease of administration also made the Denver a choice for the pilot screening. Developed in 1967, this screening test is a tool to assist health professionals in identifying potential developmental problems in young children. Widespread international use and standardization have resulted in the revised version used in the pilot study. The design of this test is for use with young children from birth to six years. The Denver II is a valuable screening tool for asymptomatic children in confirming 'intuitive suspicions with an objective measure.' Further, the tool assists in monitoring children at risk for developmental problems, specifically those who may have experienced perinatal difficulties, a problem common among children of substance abusers. The shortcomings of the Denver II were recognized as noted in several published criticisms.

The Denver II instruction manual offers cautions regarding use of the test as a predictor of future adaptive or intellectual ability or for the assignment of diagnostic labels. Suggested use of this test is as an enhancement to physical examination and diagnostic evaluation when directed. It is primarily valuable as a valid measure to compare a child's task performance to cohorts (Frankenburg et al., 1992). This study employed the Denver II to develop a standard method by which a TCC Consultant could assist sites in obtaining an organized, baseline illustration of a child's overall development and screen for any problems that could warrant a referral for specialized services.

The Denver II contains 125 items or tasks categorized to represent four areas of function or domains. These are:

1. personal-social–getting along with people and self care;
2. fine motor-adaptive–eye-to-hand coordination, manipulating small objects and problem skills;
3. language–hearing, understanding, and using language;
4. gross motor–large muscle movement.

FINDINGS

In order to appreciate the assessment procedures used for the children at the six pilot study sites, the context of the service delivery system at these sites generally, and therapeutic childcare specifically are presented. Importantly, the level of professionally educated staff, particularly at the small town and rural centers was limited at best. Moreover, there was extraordinarily high turnover, not only in administrative staff, and significantly to this paper, the direct service, therapeutic childcare staff. As noted, one of the main purposes of the study was to ascertain the level of intervention necessary with the population of children housed at these sites. One of the program expectations was that mothers gain or regain healthy parenting skills as part of the recovery process.

To that end, staff conducted an extensive case review at the six sites to understand not only the residential implications for therapeutic childcare, but also the larger treatment context for the mothers of those children. *The Nurturing Program for Families in Substance Abuse Treatment and Recovery* was chosen as the parent education model to use. This program is evidence-based, it does not require a master's level facilitator and it has an evaluation tool, the Adult and Adolescent Parenting Inventory (AAPI). Two statewide trainings were held and 125 staff from the treatment programs were trained as facilitators of the Nurturing Program. While effective as a parenting intervention, this model left out an assessment component for children. For a parenting program to be effective, a parent needs to know as much possible about their child's temperament and level of functioning.

The implementation of the Denver II also began with training of the staff to offset problems with consistency and fidelity of test administration. All sites were provided Denver materials through grant funding by the university with input from the consultant prior to clinical intervention. In preparation for support of the TCC programs, the consultant initiated conversations with the developer of the screening tool to determine if further formalized training would be required for sites. The developer indicated that use of Denver II training manual should be sufficient. The consultant offered one on one review of manual with the sites as appropriate. The consultant conducted observations of Denver assessments after training and modeled administration of screenings at two programs. Consultant technical assistance in interpretation of Denver screenings was available to all sites.

The validity and results of the screenings based upon the Consultant's efforts at the various sites was uneven. The site TCC Coordinators with strong backgrounds in childcare training, not surprisingly, proved to be the most effective in conducting the screenings. These TCC coordinators had many years in management of childcare centers and in one instance an associate's degree in early childhood development. The benefits of their experience included many years of experience observing children, skilled users of developmental screening tools, valued use of screening tools and strong community connections to agencies to support early intervention. Another important factor to ensuring the accuracy of the screening was active support from the Clinical Director of a program. Conversely, when the Clinical Director at the site was less supportive of the assessment process and subsequent services, the utility of the assessment process was compromised. Additionally, at some sites, the Director had not fully accepted the involvement of children in the treatment process as it violated tenets of "traditional" substance abuse treatment.

Fidelity in utilizing the results from scoring of the AAPI-2s was not consistent across sites. There were not good processes in place to enable feedback to parents. The Consultant encouraged that each parent have a session to discuss their results and this occurred at only two sites. Both of these sites had weekly or bi-weekly processes whereby TCC staff had parenting consult sessions with each mother. Yet, even at these two sites, there were issues. At one site, the staff had to build in time in individual counseling sessions to discuss findings from the AAPI-2 and it seemed that often the results were filed and not used. At the other site, the results were used to guide individualized goals around parent-child issues.

It is in this larger context that the Denver II was intended to be administered at the six pilot sites. Unfortunately, the programmatic issues discussed became a definite obstacle during the collection of assessment data. The consultant planned to collect Denver II data from all six of the pilot TCC sites to identify developmental issues that children present with at the time of treatment. Ultimately, the researchers obtained 23 completed Denver II tests results. Of these, 21 were administered by site staff, 1 by TCC Consultant and 1 under observation of TCC Consultant. There were more children in residence during the study period with their mothers than these numbers reflect, but the problems discussed precluded completing more.

Of the 23 children screened using the Denver II in this study, there were 14 girls and 9 boys. Seventeen children were Caucasian, five were African American and one was biracial. The range age in months of the children screened was 2 to 69. The median age was 30 months with a mean age of 34 months.

Of the 23 children screened, 13 or 57% presented with a variety of developmental difficulties. Ten children, or 43% were at a typical level of development. Specific developmental problems were identified as follows:

personal-social–4 children or 17%
fine motor-adaptive–6 children or 26%
language–8 children or 35%
gross motor–3 children or 13%

By way of comparison, Simpson, Colpe, and Greenspan (2003), utilizing data from the 1994-95 National Health Interview Survey for Disabilities (NHIS-D) of 15,000 children, found that only 3.3% had functional delays (FD) and 3.4% had general delays (GD). However, they found that only 17% of the children with FD and 31% of those with GD were receiving special services. Moreover, they found that children with both FD and GD were more likely to be male and to be living in families with incomes below 200% of the poverty level. They suggest that large national surveys may be underestimating the percentage of children with developmental delays. Based upon the assessments done at the residential sites, and despite the obstacles, intervention actions increased. On the other hand, sites were clearly at differing levels in their ability to identify and secure services to address the developmental needs of children in need of early intervention services. On a case by case basis, actions commenced. For example, the TCC Consultant recommended re-screening prior to discharge for one child who was born on site and whose mother was near discharge. The TCC Consultant recommended that the discharge plan for this child include referral to early intervention services. Four children were identified as receiving no services for identified delays. Two of these cases involved children whose mothers left treatment against medical advice. One of these children was placed in foster care. For one child, the time from Denver II screening and chart audit was too short for site to have developed treatment plan. The final child had a medical condition that could potentially be cause for gross motor delays. Suggestions were made to site TCC staff to share Denver II findings with mother to develop an appropriate plan with child's pediatrician.

Seven children were referred to community agencies for early intervention services to include full developmental evaluations. Of these seven, two were not receiving services at the conclusion of this study's evaluation period. Physical therapy had begun for one child and speech therapy had begun for four children. The local school system had been notified to complete a full evaluation for one child.

DISCUSSION

Although the Denver II data gathered in this study is very preliminary, it appears that a majority of the population of children at the sites studied this year do have a variety of developmental deficits. Given that over half the children screened in these sites have some type of developmental delay, it highlights the need to insure that young children are properly evaluated.

Additionally, the findings of this study can provide guidance for treatment plans for children in the residential treatment centers to include early intervention services as partners in the treatment program. Further analysis of pretest/posttest Denver II data could be useful to help sites evaluate the effectiveness of developmental interventions.

Also noted, some of the sites struggled to integrate developmental screening into their assessment process for children. These problems appeared to be related to lack of staff, delays in becoming adapted to new procedures, staff turnover, getting training to staff, and lack of using written training resources. Given the apparent need for services, TCC providers will be challenged to overcome some of these obstacles and develop strategies that help bring these services to the children.

In reviewing the sites' current intervention approaches, it becomes clear that some sites have been able to successfully access community agencies that provide developmental services for the children whereas others experienced delays and/or a lack of service. Some sites are in the process of setting up protocols that will enable them to strengthen collaboration with agencies to access existing developmental data or provide developmental assessment for the children in their care.

CONCLUSION

In summary, while sites struggle with a variety of barriers, developmental services appear necessary for children residing with mother's in residential treatment. However, regardless of the quality of the assessment tool, there must be a commitment and agreement from site staff that the children are a part of the treatment regimen. Only then can the fidelity of the assessment tools be protected.

Therefore, if programs are going to offer mothers the opportunity to have their children in treatment with them there needs to be staff cross training to prepare for the dual focus of the treatment community as well as individual assessment and treatment protocols for the children.

REFERENCES

Baker, P. & Carson, A. (1999). I take care of my kids: Mothering practices of substance abusing women. *Gender and Society, 13*(3), 347-363.

—— (2001). Child care services for children in out-of-home care. Casey Family Programs. Washington D. C.

Child Care Early Education Research Center. National Center for Children and Poverty. http://www.childcareresearch.org/discover/index.jsp

Clark, W. H. (2001). Residential substance abuse treatment for pregnant and post-partum women and their children. *Child Welfare, 80*(2), 179-198.

Connors, N. A., Bradley, R. H., & Whiteside-Mansell, L. (2001). A comprehensive substance abuse treatment program for women and their children: An initial evaluation. *Journal of Substance Abuse Treatment, 21*(2), 67-75.

Frankenburg, W. K., Dodds, J., Archer, P., Shapiro, H., & Bresnick, B. (1992). The Denver II: A major revision and restandardization of the developmental screening test. *Pediactrics, 89*(1), 91-97.

Grella, C. E., Joshi, V., & Hser, Y. I. (2000). Program variation in treatment outcomes among women in residential drug treatment. *Evaluation Review, 24*(4), 364-383.

Jackson, M. (1995). Afrocentric treatment of African American women and their children in residential chemical dependency programs. *Journal of Black Studies, 26*(1), 17-30.

Knight, D. K., Logan, S. M., & Simpson, D. P. (2001). Predictors of program completion for women in residential substance abuse treatment. *The American Journal of Drug and Alcohol Abuse, 27*(1), 1-18.

Metsch, L. R., Rivers, J. E., Miller, M., Bohs, R., & McCoy, C. B. (1995). Implementation of a family centered treatment program for substance abusing women and their children. *Journal of Psychoactive Drugs, 27*(1), 73-83.

Moore, E., Armsden, G., & Gogerty, P. L. (1998). Twelve year follow-up study of maltreated and at-risk children who received early therapeutic childcare. *Child Maltrement, 3*(1), 3-16.

Scott-Lennox, J., Rose, R., Bohleg, A., & Lennox, R. (2000). The impact of women's family status on completion of substance abuse treatment. *Journal of Behavioral Health Services and Research, 27*(4), 366-379.

Simpson, G., Colpe, L., & Greenspan, S. (2003). Measuring functional developmental delay in infants and young children: prevalence rates the NHIS-D. *Pediatric Perinatal Epidemiology, 17*(1), 68-80.

Taylor and Francis. (2004). Children of mothers with serious substance abuse problems: An accumulation of research. *The American Journal of Substance Abuse, 30*(1),

Uziel-Miller, N. D. & Lyons, J. S. (2000). Specialized substance abuse treatment for women and their children: An analysis of program design. *Journal of Substance Abuse Treatment, 19*(4), 355-367.

Assessing Youth Strengths in a Residential Juvenile Correctional Program

William H. Barton, PhD
Juliette R. Mackin, PhD
Jerrold Fields, MSW

INTRODUCTION

This article describes the implementation and early results of adopting a strengths-based assessment in a residential juvenile correctional program. In response to a series of incidents and critical reports regarding practices at the Johnson Youth Center Treatment Unit (JYCTU) (Heafner, 2006a, 2006b), a secure juvenile correctional program in Juneau, the Alaska Division of Juvenile Justice (DJJ) initiated efforts to transform the culture of the institution into a less punitive environment. A major element of the transformation involved the JYCTU supplementing its usual assessments of offense characteristics and social history with an assessment of youth strengths to enable staff to learn about the youths' particular strengths; form deeper, more positive relationships with them; and develop richer, more individualized service plans. The instrument selected, the Youth Competency Assessment (YCA), was developed specifically for use in juvenile justice settings by a research team and advisory committee headed by staff at NPC Research (Mackin, Weller, Tarte, & Nissen, 2005; Nissen, Mackin, Weller, & Tarte, 2005). This article describes the first known attempt to apply the YCA in a secure residential correctional setting.

Since the founding of the first juvenile court in Chicago in 1899, the juvenile justice system has struggled with balancing its goals of protecting public safety and providing for the best interests of the child (Bernard, 1992). Trends in juvenile justice policy and practice have alternated between punitive and rehabilitative responses to young offenders (Bernard, 1992; Howell, 2003). In the 1990s, "get tough" responses resulted in many states lowering the maximum age of juvenile court jurisdiction (to enable more youths' cases to be processed in adult court), transferring certain juvenile offenders to the adult system via legislative mandate or prosecutorial discretion, enacting "three strikes" and "zero tolerance" policies, and imposing longer terms of confinement (Snyder & Sickmund, 2006). Despite the decline in juvenile crime rates during the last decade, pre-adjudicatory detention and post-adjudicatory residential placements remain over-used, largely ineffective in reducing recidivism, and plagued with overcrowding and deplorable conditions (Abrams, 2005; Cannon,

2004; Lerner, 1986; Lispsey, 1992; Parent et al., 1994; Snyder & Sickmund, 2006; Steinberg, Chung, & Little, 2004).

More recently, however, the field has seen a resurgence of optimism that correctional treatment can be effective for adults and juveniles, but only if it follows certain principles such as those described by Andrews and colleagues (Andrews, 1995; Andrews & Bonta, 1998; Andrews et al., 1990). Such principles build upon accumulated research that has identified specific risk factors associated with increased probability of youth problem behaviors and protective factors that prevent or buffer exposure to such risks (Hawkins, Catalano, & Miller, 1992; Hawkins et al., 2000; Lipsey & Derzon, 1998; Lipsey & Wilson, 1998). Effective interventions address specific risks and needs, are behaviorally focused, target high risk offenders, and are delivered in ways compatible with the individual learning style of offenders (Andrews, 1995; Andrews & Bonta, 1998; Andrews et al., 1990). Compendia of evidence-based programs, that is, those with demonstrated effectiveness in preventing or reducing recidivism among juvenile offenders, have emerged (Aos, Phipps, Barnoski, & Lieb, 2001; Mihalic, Fagan, Irwin, Ballard, & Elliott, 2004; Office of Juvenile Justice and Delinquency Prevention, n.d.; Sherman et al., 1997). Yet, even evidence-based treatment models view youth through a "deficit-based" lens, analogous to the medical model in which problems can be diagnosed and treatments delivered to fix the problems or at least attenuate symptoms.

Many young people in correctional settings may indeed have mental health issues; some estimate that as many as 70% of youths in detention or residential programs meet the criteria for at least one such condition (Teplin, Abram, McClelland, Dulcan, & Mericle, 2002; Wasserman, Ko, & McReynolds, 2004). Certainly such needs should be addressed. But, by simply focusing on needs and risks, programs may be missing a crucial opportunity to promote more basic positive youth development by taking a more holistic view of youth, which includes risks, needs *and* strengths in ways that may greatly enhance the youths' long-term prospects for successful life outcomes.

To capitalize on that opportunity, juvenile justice practitioners might benefit from more explicitly adopting strengths-based, positive youth development principles. Proponents of positive youth development note that being "problem free isn't fully prepared" (Pittman & Irby, 1996, p. 3). In other words, simply reducing youths' engagement in problem behaviors is no guarantee that they are thus equipped with the skills and attitudes needed to lead independent, healthy, and productive lives. Of course, the juvenile justice system cannot and should not abandon its goals of protecting public safety and providing treatment to help youth address problem areas. But the system could also pursue more universal goals of positive youth development (competence, character, connections, confidence, and contribution, as described by Hamilton, Hamilton, & Pittman, 2004). Moreover, focusing on strengths and positive youth development goals may increase youth accountability by helping them become more engaged in and attached to conventional society. Thus, by adopting this perspective, juvenile justice programs may be able to promote long-term, healthy development while doing an even better job of preventing subsequent problem behaviors than by relying on addressing only risks and needs.

To effectively and consistently pursue positive youth development goals, staff in juvenile justice settings first need to view the youth in their care not as dangerous individuals to be controlled or as sick individuals to be treated, but as young people with strengths, interests, and dreams who can be encouraged to build upon those characteristics in positive ways. Such a strengths-based approach (Rapp, 1998; Saleebey, 2002) is becoming more common in mental health and child welfare settings but is still relatively rare in juvenile or criminal justice settings. Several researchers and practitioners, however, have advocated its potential applicability to such settings (Butts, Mayer, & Cusick, 2005; Clark, 1997, 1998; Franz, 1994, 2001; Maruna & LeBel, 2003; Northey, Primer, & Christensen, 1997; Van Wormer, 1999). A strengths-based approach begins with the assumptions that all people have strengths within themselves and in their environment (families and communities) and that change is more likely to occur when the individual is engaged as an active partner in the process of setting goals and choosing action strategies (Cowger & Snively, 2002; Rapp, 1998; Saleebey, 2002). It follows, then, that a juvenile justice program electing to adopt a strengths-based approach will need to modify its assessment procedures to include the systematic identification of youths' strengths.

There is a long history of assessments in juvenile justice settings. Assessments in residential juvenile correctional programs have often been used to establish typologies of youth to guide placement decisions, security levels, and treatment programming. For example, the California Youth Authority developed a system of classification based on youths' interpersonal maturity levels (I-levels) to assign placements and differential intervention strategies (Warren et al., 1966). Other assessment tools used in juvenile justice settings include inventories of mental health concerns, such as the Massachusetts Youth Screening Instrument, Second Version (MAYSI-2), developed by Grisso and Barnum (2000). Many juvenile justice agencies and programs use assessments derived from theories of criminogenic needs (Andrews et al., 1990), that is, factors that research has shown are correlated with offending behaviors. Examples include the Youth Level of Services/Case Management Inventory (YLS/CMI) (Hoge & Andrews, 1996), the Washington State Juvenile Court Assessment (Barnoski, 2004), and the Oregon JCP Assessment (NPC Research, 2006). The most recent versions of these tools include some items related to strengths or protective factors, but are primarily oriented towards identifying risks to be controlled or reduced through supervision, custody level, or interventions, and needs to be addressed in the treatment plan through referrals to specialized services.

Strengths-based assessments are both a tool and a process. They are different from risk and needs assessments in that they collect additional content (e.g., strengths, interests, supports, potential) as well as meet additional objectives. Beyond determining risk to re-offend and identifying unmet needs, strengths-based assessments build rapport and engagement. Staff can develop stronger, positive relationships with the youth (and their families) and develop more individualized case plans. For example, if a youth is especially interested or talented in art or music, the case plan can include enhancing those talents and even include opportunities for the youth to produce artistic works or performances while in the program, perhaps even in the community outside of the facility. Or, the case plan could provide opportunities for that youth to tutor or mentor others with similar interests but less proficiency, again, either within the facility or the community. For another example, if a youth is interested in computer games, that interest could be built upon and broadened to other computer applications. The Youth Competency Assessment, to be described in more detail in the next section, is a strengths-based assessment protocol developed specifically for use in juvenile justice, and is the tool adopted by the JYCTU. It must be emphasized that the use of the YCA or other strengths-based assessment tool is intended to supplement the more traditional assessment protocols, not to replace them.

There is as yet little empirical evidence of the effectiveness or viability of strengths-based, positive youth development principles in juvenile justice settings. Clearly, the contrasting organizational cultures of traditional juvenile justice settings and the strengths-based perspective suggest potential challenges to implementation of the latter, particularly in secure, residential programs (Barton, 2004, 2006; Schwartz, 2001; Torbet & Thomas, 2005). The recent effort of the JYCTU to adopt a strengths-based approach is thus noteworthy. Although it is too soon to assess the effects on youth outcomes, marked changes in the culture of the organization are already apparent. The next sections discuss the development of the YCA; the prior problematic context of the JYCTU; the introduction of the YCA to this setting; and some immediate results in terms of more individualized case planning, changes in the organizational environment, and staff perceptions of the changes. The JYCTU experience to date provides lessons for other juvenile correctional institutions regarding the potential benefits and challenges of adopting a more strengths-based approach.

THE YOUTH COMPETENCY ASSESSMENT

The Youth Competency Assessment is a strengths-based assessment tool and protocol for professionals working with youth and their families. It was developed for use in juvenile justice settings, as well as for substance abuse treatment providers and community treatment or intervention programs. NPC Research, in Portland, Oregon, developed and tested the YCA tool and process through a grant from The Robert Wood Johnson Foundation, in collaboration with staff from three Oregon county juvenile departments.

The YCA was developed to help juvenile justice and adolescent treatment systems incorporate strengths into their assessment and service planning processes. This instrument was not designed to replace existing risk or problem identification tools, but rather to expand, strengthen, and improve a service system's capacity to include the positive elements of a youth, the youth's family, peers, and/or community in a well-balanced assessment and service profile. The YCA provides a foundation on which to build healthy youth and strong families, and a structure in which to create new types of service plans that amplify and encourage the development of positive, pro-social behaviors. It is based on the theoretical foundations of balanced and restorative justice (e.g., Bazemore & Umbreit, 1994), strength-based approaches to service delivery (e.g., Saleebey, 2002), moral development (e.g., Berkowitz & Grych, 1998), adolescent development (e.g., Steinberg & Morris, 2001), and sense of community (e.g., Perkins, Florin, Rich, Wandersman, & Chavis, 1990), among others.

The tool and protocol help staff meet the following three goals:

1. Ensure accountability and promote public safety, through enhancing youths' moral development
   - Support efforts to repair harm
   - Use mistakes and past negative behavior and choices as learning opportunities
2. Provide mechanisms for youth to develop a healthy identity
   - Encourage involvements in pro-social activities and develop career interests
3. Connect youth to community, family, and peers
   - Build on or identify positive mentoring opportunities and develop positive relationships
   - Identify and generate resources to support the youth and help her/him be successful

The YCA is a set of open-ended questions asked as a conversational, informal in-person interview between a staff person and a youth. The materials can also be used with a parent or guardian present or adapted to use with the caregiver alone. The questions help build rapport, trust, and respect between the staff and youth, developing a relationship that is the foundation of engaging the youth and family in the service plan and in behavior change. The short form of the YCA may be found in Appendix A.

Pilot Testing

NPC Research developed the YCA tool and process with the assistance of a national panel of experts in the areas of juvenile justice, restorative justice, adolescent treatment, and psychometrics. Youth were involved in the development of the assessment questions and format. The research team pilot tested the training curriculum, tool, and process in three different communities and engaged a local advisory panel of juvenile justice staff and administrators who consulted with the developers on every aspect of the project. Focus groups of staff using the tool also provided feedback. Suggestions from these various groups of experts contributed to improvements in the training materials and tool, and development of implementation guidelines for other sites. While additional studies need to be conducted to collect and analyze youth-level outcome data and long-term system change data, the tool in its current form has face and content validity and seems to be measuring the constructs of interest.

Benefits of the YCA

Staff using the tool reported improved rapport with and increased buy-in from youth and their parents/guardians, increased job satisfaction, and increased staff morale. They also reported cases ending more quickly and decreased need for the use of sanctions. Youth reported increased positive perceptions of the juvenile justice staff, including feeling as though their points of view were taken into account and that what they did wrong was not the focus of their meetings. The YCA increased strengths-based practice and improved the use of positive non-verbal cues and positive atmosphere of interviews with youth and their families, based on coded videotapes of assessments conducted by staff using the YCA compared to staff using traditional assessment tools (Mackin, Weller, & Tarte, 2004).

Dissemination Through Training

The research team compiled a list of lessons learned through the pilot study, which have been used to enhance training and provide implementation strategies for subsequent sites. The research team and juvenile department staff partners have offered trainings at national conferences and through various professional organizations. The training materials and the tools are public domain and available on-line for use or adaptation by any interested organization or individual. In addition, staff from the research team and pilot sites have been hired to conduct trainings for juvenile justice and social services staff in other locations. The intent of the team is to share the philosophy of incorporating a strength-based approach into work with youth and families, and to provide tools for enhancing risk and needs assessment and developing more holistic, culturally responsive, and individualized service plans.

THE PATH TOWARDS CHANGE
AT THE JYC TREATMENT UNIT

The Johnson Youth Center (JYC), operated by the Alaska Division of Juvenile Justice (DJJ) in Juneau, houses juvenile probation services, an 8-bed secure detention center, and a 20-bed secure treatment unit. The treatment unit (JYCTU) was added in 1999, and is located in a separate building at the rear of the complex. Staffing in the treatment unit consists of a Superintendent (who also administers the detention unit), Treatment Unit Supervisor, Mental Health Counselor, three floor supervisors and seven line staff. Other staff (teachers, medical staff, etc.) serve both the detention and treatment units. The facility houses males between the ages of 15 and 18 who have been adjudicated for a variety of moderate to serious offenses such as assault, theft, robbery, arson, burglary and misconduct involving controlled substances (Heafner, 2006a). In fiscal year 2006 the treatment unit's average daily population was 16 and the average length of stay was 13 months. Approximately half of the youth were Alaska Native, 39% were Caucasian, and 11% were African American.

The Previous Culture of the JYCTU

During the early years of the JYCTU, lengths of stay were relatively long (yearly averages were between 11 and 13 months), and this enabled the program to provide residents the opportunity to spend time transitioning back into the community. This reentry period included participating in community work service activities and off-unit activities. There was a positive approach to developing partnerships with outside community agencies, including a program serving youth with developmental disabilities, a horse stable, and extensive use of volunteers, including foster grand parenting, churches, and 12-step programs, to establish mentoring and community supports for youth leaving the facility.

Although the program was referred to as a treatment facility, prior to 2006 the JYCTU emphasized its correctional role. Leadership appeared to adopt a hands-off approach; there was very little mentoring of staff. The program staff developed initial policies and procedures, rules, and a level system focused primarily on safety, security, and behavioral management. With a correctional culture that tended towards being punitive, staff were not trained to focus on developing positive relationships with the youth. This contributed to reports of an "us versus them" dynamic on the unit between staff and residents. Staff and residents perceived the unit climate/environment as being tense, with both groups anticipating crises/eruptions. This tension also contributed to numerous reports of poor relationships, a general lack of respect, and a lack of trust between youth and staff, resulting in acting out behaviors and rigid/reactive staff responses, such as confining youth to their rooms or taking away points or privileges. This cycle confirmed the fears and beliefs of both residents and staff about the other group.

The residents' thoughts, feelings, and perspectives were often discounted and treatment goals were established with minimal participation from residents and their families. The goals were generally problem oriented and uniform (or standard) across youth, regardless of their individual needs and interests. Case planning meetings did not occur on a regular basis and when they did, they commonly did not include input from the youth or their families.

During this period, the program did not have a full-time mental health professional and relied on outside contractors, including a psychiatrist, psychologist, and clinicians from various community agencies. There was very little emphasis on clinical oversight and supervision. Few residents received consistent professional mental health treatment including individual, family, or group therapy. Treatment groups were sporadic and informational or educational rather than therapeutic.

Moving Towards Change

DJJ leadership hired a new Superintendent for JYC in late 2005 with the goal of significantly improving both the facility's culture and programming. The Division sent a veteran Program Coordinator as a consultant to provide on-site assessment and technical assistance. After a weeklong site visit, this consultant produced two reports, the first outlining an extensive array of concerns regarding policies and practices at the JYC (Heafner, 2006a), and the second containing a series of recommendations for improvement and an action plan (Heafner, 2006b). Problems identified included insufficient assessments, inconsistent quality of documentation in case files, lack of formalized training in case management, and the absence of a system of graduated sanctions and incentives. In addition, although the program had developed some reentry transition and community partnerships, they were not as effective or comprehensive as they could have been (Heafner, 2006a). Underlying the many specific recommendations was a mandate for a system-wide transformation of the culture of the facility into a strengths-based environment, providing comprehensive, individualized assessment and case planning, and developing additional linkages with the community (Heafner, 2006b). The action plan included adopting the YCA, and the Division contracted with the Northwest Professional Consortium (NPC Research) to provide the training.[1]

Introducing the YCA at the JYCTU

JYCTU staff received training in the use of the YCA in September 2006. The training team consisted of the lead researcher from the YCA pilot project and a juvenile court counselor from one of the pilot sites.

This team brought the theoretical background of the tool and approach, experience with the development and implementation of the instrument, and expertise in juvenile justice research, combined with the direct service, clinical experience of a staff person who had used the YCA and other strength-based practices, both in residential and intake settings. The combination of research and practice helped provide credibility of the tool and process to managers and staff at the JYCTU. The training was attended by JYC staff, community partner agency representatives, the state juvenile justice researcher, and state Division leadership.

The training began with local and state staff describing the plans and vision for the training and the implementation of the YCA at the JYCTU. It then engaged staff in a variety of exercises and discussions. The researcher presented an overview of the strengths perspective and approach, and why it is beneficial and appropriate for juvenile justice agencies. Staff practiced drawing out strengths and analyzing a case example, and discussed incorporating a strength-based frame of reference into their work. They finished the first day by returning to the facility to practice using the YCA with youth on the unit. The second day of training focused on applying information from the YCA to case planning and management, using creative approaches to connecting with community resources, anticipating challenges, and generating strategies for how to overcome them. The day ended with a discussion of concrete plans for implementation, task assignments, and establishment of timelines.

PRELIMINARY RESULTS

Now, about 6 months after the introduction of the YCA and the strengths-based approach at the JYCTU, several changes are apparent, as will be detailed in this section. Formal policies and procedures have been modified, a new approach to practice has been instituted, incidents and complaints have been reduced, and a measurable change in the social climate of the institution is evident. Not all the changes have been uniformly positive, as the transformation has prompted the resignation of several veteran treatment unit staff.

Revisions to Unit Policies and Procedures

The introduction of a strengths-based perspective to the Treatment program required the revision of numerous Johnson Youth Center Policies and Procedures (JYC P&P) and a reevaluation of unit practices. Listed below are a few examples of the changes that have taken place.

- Revised JYC P&P Treatment Unit admissions process to reflect the inclusion of strengths-based language in the letter sent to families when the residents are admitted to the program.
- Changed procedures for admitting youth to the Treatment Unit by assigning Treatment Teams and administering the YCA prior to a resident being transferred to the Unit.
- Revised JYC P&P regarding the discipline process to reflect a strengths-based approach to addressing poor behavior by residents both on and off facility grounds. For example, instead of using room confinement or secure isolation, a strengths-based approach incorporates de-escalation counseling and the building of positive relationships to prevent crisis situations and to help mitigate crisis situations that do occur.
- Revised the point system allowing youth to earn and maintain privileges on the Unit to ensure that residents *earn* rather than *lose* points each day and that their progress is reviewed at least once per shift during a group points meeting.
- Revised JYC P&P addressing resident passes away from the facility to recognize that effective transition programming requires what Altschuler and Armstrong (1991) call "testing and probing" a youth's reintegration into the community. Rather than being seen as simply a privilege to be earned or withheld based upon behavior in the Unit, passes provide the resident opportunities to practice the skills learned on the Treatment Unit while in the community. Upon the resident's return from the community, staff and the youth engage in a strengths-based debriefing to discuss the positive and negative aspects of the experience in the community. When setbacks are encountered (e.g., failing to return from a pass or failed urinalysis tests upon return to the facility), staff are expected to address these concerns by first looking at recent accomplishments or any improvement over past setbacks, then looking towards increasing resources (e.g., individual counseling or groups), rather than employing punitive measures, to shape future behavior.

Adopting Strengths-Based Practices

The Youth Competency Assessment has been used with 27 residents of the JYCTU since its introduction to the program. A strengths-based focus starts when a youth has been accepted to the JYCTU and is in pre-admission on the detention unit. At this point, a staff member is assigned to interview the youth using the YCA. In conjunction with this assessment, the clinician interviews the parent(s)/guardian, also using the YCA as part of the interview, for incorporation into the clinical assessment. The information from the parent(s)/guardian and the youth, along with information about risks and needs based on the YLS/CMI, are included in the development of an initial treatment plan. The youth and parent(s)/guardian are then fully involved in developing treatment goals that are individualized, strengths-based, and have a focus on transitional planning for the youth's return into the community. Subsequent meetings occur monthly between the assigned staff person and the youth in order to review progress toward goals, adjust the plan, or establish new goals as needed.

Staff report greater openness to including creative or innovative strategies in treatment plans. If an idea seems feasible to implement and does not compromise the safety of the resident or the community, it is now being considered. In addition, staff devote greater attention to involving community partners and other support persons identified by the resident or family members in supporting the plan, especially in assisting towards transitional planning and aftercare. Transition plans are being developed earlier than in the past. These transition plans are strengths-based, and include connecting the youth with supports within the community and having the youth spend more time in the community. As a result of this earlier, more thorough transition planning, lengths of stays have become shorter, decreasing from the previous years' averages of 11-13 months to 9 months for youth released so far in fiscal year 2007.

Decrease in Incidents and Complaints

As discussed previously, the prior culture at the JYCTU could be characterized as relatively punitive. Unfortunately, JYC records of incidents and complaints prior to the arrival of the new superintendent in late 2005 are unreliable. Since then, however, record keeping has improved. Thus it is possible to compare the frequency of incidents and complaints for several months prior to the introduction of the strengths-based approach (January to mid-September of 2006) with those during the first few months after implementation (mid-September 2006, through March 2007). Table 1 presents this comparison. It is clear that there have been considerably fewer critical incidents and complaints since the introduction of the strengths-based approach. In the

TABLE 1. Critical Incidents at the JYCTU Pre- and Post-YCA Training

Type of Incident	Pre-YCA 1/1/06-9/19/06	Post-YCA 9/20/06-3/31/07
Resident on resident assault	4	1
Resident verbal outburst directed towards staff/failure to follow staff instructions	12	3
Resident verbal threats of physical harm against staff	5	0
Resident physical restraint (involving two or more staff)	3	1
Resident self harm behaviors (hitting / kicking walls and doors, self mutilation, suicide gestures)	4	1
Resident alcohol or drug use while on pass from the facility	2	1
Resident escape planning	1	0
Contraband on unit (any items not approved for residents in the treatment program manual)	9	1
Telephonic complaints received by the Superintendent re: staff and/or services from residents' family members	14	0
Written complaints to the DJJ state offices	2	0
Resident escapes from pass	1	2
Total	57	10
Number of months in period	9.5	6.5
Incidents per month	6.7	1.5

pre-YCA period, there was an average of 6.7 incidents or complaints per month compared with only 1.5 per month in the post-YCA period. Especially noteworthy have been the reductions in complaints from residents' families, youths' verbal or physical outbursts, and youths' bringing contraband of any kind onto the Unit. The only category showing a post-YCA increase is escapes from passes (from 1 to 2), perhaps an outgrowth of the more frequent use of passes in conjunction with more comprehensive transition planning.

Social Climate Changes at the JYCTU

To assess the social climate of the facility, the JYCTU used the Correctional Institutions Environment Scale (CIES) developed by Moos (1974, 1987). The CIES, which has been widely used in both juvenile and adult correctional settings, was completed by youth and staff in early September 2006, prior to the YCA training, and again in March

2007. The CIES contains nine subscales covering three dimensions, defined as follows:

Relational Dimension

- *Involvement*–how active residents are in the day-to-day functioning of the program.
- *Support*–the extent to which residents are encouraged to help and support other residents; how supportive the staff is toward residents.
- *Expressiveness*–how much the program encourages the open expression of feelings by residents and staff.

Personal Growth Dimension

- *Autonomy*–the extent to which residents are encouraged to take initiative in planning activities and to take leadership in the unit.
- *Practical orientation*–the degree to which residents learn practical skills and are prepared for release from the program.
- *Personal problem orientation*–the extent to which residents are encouraged to understand their personal problems and feelings.

System Maintenance Dimension

- *Order and organization*–how important order and organization are in the program.
- *Clarity*–the extent to which residents know what to expect in the day-to-day routine of the program and the explicitness of rules and procedures.
- *Staff control*–the degree to which staff use measures to keep residents under necessary controls. (Moos, 1987)

Each scale has either 9 or 10 true-false items, with item wording varied so that some "true" responses and some "false" responses reflect positive perceptions of the climate dimension. For scoring purposes, each response reflecting a positive perception is counted. Scores on each of the scales can range from 0 to either 9 or 10, with higher scores reflecting more positive climate aspects.[2] The CIES has been normed on large samples of residents and staff in juvenile and adult correctional institutions across the United States.

Social climate change at the JYCTU was assessed by comparing the baseline CIES scale scores with those obtained 6 months after the introduction of the YCA. Although the groups of residents and staff completing the scales at the two times contained some of the same individuals, most were different, and the anonymity of responses prevented linking of individual pre- and post-YCA scores in any event. Therefore, independent t-tests were performed. Furthermore, since the introduction of the YCA and the strengths-based practices was intended to improve the climate of the institution, one-tail tests of significance were used.[3] The results of these t-tests are shown in Tables 2 (for residents) and 3 (for staff).

All youth residents currently placed in the Treatment Unit at the time of each administration completed the CIES (17 in September 2006; 13 in March 2007). Residents' perceptions suggest that the climate at the JYCTU had improved considerably 6 months after the introduction of the YCA. They reported significantly higher levels of support, expressiveness, autonomy, practical orientation, and clarity. Although not reaching statistical significance, scores on the remaining four scales were also slightly higher at the 6-month follow-up. Note that the relatively small number of respondents provides little statistical power for these analyses, that is, in order to be statistically significant, the difference between the means would have to be quite large. In this context, finding significant changes on five of the nine subscales is impressive. Compared with CIES normative samples (Moos, 1987), the JYCTU residents' baseline

TABLE 2. Social Climate Pre- and Post-YCA: Residents

CIES Subscale (No. of Items)	Pre-YCA (9/06) N = 17		Post-YCA (3/07) N = 13		
	Mean	Std. Dev.	Mean	Std. Dev.	t
Involvement (10)	2.88	1.87	4.15	2.13	1.678
Support (10)	4.12	2.19	6.38	2.36	2.624**
Expressiveness (9)	2.82	1.89	4.46	1.50	2.480**
Autonomy (9)	3.82	1.72	4.92	1.14	1.927*
Practical Orientation (10)	5.82	2.12	7.46	1.71	2.199*
Personal Problem Orientation (9)	2.82	1.76	3.69	1.80	1.282
Order and Organization (10)	5.00	2.06	6.38	2.29	1.679
Clarity (10)	4.35	2.08	5.85	1.87	1.966*
Staff Control (9)	5.94	1.47	6.31	2.17	0.532

* p < .05; ** p < .01; df = 28, one-tailed.

TABLE 3. Social Climate Pre- and Post-YCA: Staff[a]

CIES Subscale (No. of Items)	Pre-YCA (9/06) N = 9		Post-YCA (3/07) N = 12		
	Mean	Std. Dev.	Mean	Std. Dev.	t
Involvement (10)	4.22	2.66	5.17	2.56	0.782
Support (10)	7.00	2.21	8.00	1.21	1.261
Expressiveness (9)	3.00	1.83	4.50	1.43	2.007*
Autonomy (9)	4.11	1.73	7.00	1.46	3.941**
Practical Orientation (10)	7.33	2.21	9.00	0.98	2.210*
Personal Problem Orientation (9)	5.00	2.54	5.50	1.48	0.539
Order and Organization (10)	5.56	2.45	5.83	2.52	0.240
Clarity (10)	5.44	1.83	5.50	2.46	0.054
Staff Control (9)	5.44	1.42	4.75	1.30	−1.107

* $p < .05$; ** $p < .01$; df = 19, one-tailed.
[a] No female staff completed the Pre-YCA CIES. The Post-YCA staff respondents included 4 female staff. Analyses excluding the female staff showed the same pattern of results.

scores were below the norm on all but one subscale (order and organization); at follow-up, their scores were above the norms on all subscales except involvement and personal problem orientation.

Nine staff members completed the CIES in September 2006; 12 completed it at the March 2007 follow-up. Their results corroborated those of the residents, with higher scale scores at follow-up on all but one dimension (staff control), although only three of the differences were statistically significant (on expressiveness, autonomy, and practical orientation). That residents also reported significant improvements on these subscales adds validity to the results. JYCTU staff scores at baseline were below the CIES norm on all but one subscale (staff control); at follow-up their scores were above the norm on three subscales (support, autonomy, and practical orientation).

Staff Turnover

The Treatment Unit operates with a total of 14 full-time, permanent positions. Since the YCA training, the turnover rate has been 50 percent. The Treatment Unit Supervisor transferred to the Detention Unit in October 2006. One Juvenile Justice Officer transferred and five resigned between October 2006 and April 2007. Such extensive turnover creates problems associated with finding and training new staff, places a burden on remaining staff while positions are temporarily un-filled, and causes disruption for the youth. On the other hand, staff turn-over also presents an opportunity to replace those who may have been wedded to the former ways of doing business with others who may be more suited to the new, strengths-based perspective.

DISCUSSION

Prior to the introduction of strengths-based perspective training and the use of the YCA, treatment goal development and case planning at the JYCTU were widely characterized as deficit-based. Delinquent acts in the community and poor behaviors in educational and institutional settings were the focus of the goals and strategies outlined during the first 30 days on the Treatment Unit, and the resulting case planning re-ports reflected this orientation. Resident and parental/guardian partici-pation in this process was minimal or non-existent; as a result, any collaboration efforts attempted between JYCTU treatment teams and families during the extended term treatment process met with a limited degree of success. Assertions from residents and families that the treat-ment program resembled a "corrections" or "prison" environment were common prior to the training. In turn, JYCTU staff reported a lack of safety and job satisfaction on the Unit due to the number of verbal out-bursts by angry residents, threats of physical harm, and the combative restraints they were required to employ while on duty.

Adopting a strengths-based approach has ushered in a new era at the JYCTU. Many changes in the Treatment Unit have occurred, such as:

- Updating and clarifying the rulebook and policy and procedures;
- Developing a curriculum-based approach inclusive of consistent and well thought out treatment groups;
- Supporting newly developed in-house clinical services;
- Providing staff training to support a strengths-based, case manage-ment role versus a correctional role;
- Providing hands-on leadership;
- Further enhancing transitional services, including supporting pre-existing partnerships and developing new partnerships; and
- Removing many punitive approaches used in the past while at the same time maintaining an emphasis on safety and security.

The strengths-based approach has provided an excellent foundation for line staff in shifting to a case management role, especially in regards to initial treatment planning and case planning meetings. The other noticeable enhancement in services is that staff now spends more time interacting with the residents rather than directing them.

Bringing the notion of strengths front and center in the assessment and case planning process has served as the catalyst for a more profound culture change in the facility. The early results are highly promising. There has been a marked decline in critical incidents and complaints in the months following the training, and significant improvements in several aspects of the social climate have been observed. Although not all of the original treatment unit staff embraced the new perspective, as evidenced by high turnover, leadership at JYC and DJJ remains committed to the transformation process. DJJ has also decided to bring strengths-based perspective/YCA training to another facility in the state. As one senior DJJ administrator commented, "What's going on at JYC is the spark igniting discussions at the Division level regarding moving the entire state system in this direction" (James Heafner, personal communication, 3/5/07).

It is possible that many of the positive changes observed at the JYCTU resulted from the introduction of new staff or the presence of a different group of residents rather than from the implementation of the YCA and the strengths perspective per se. It is also possible that the changes reflect a short-term "honeymoon" period that may erode over time. Moreover, it is still too early to assess whether the changes will make it more likely that the youth will experience long-term benefits in terms of productive citizenship and reduced recidivism. Despite such caveats, the experience of the JYCTU demonstrates that it is possible to introduce a strengths-based perspective even in the traditionally punitive context of a secure juvenile correctional setting.

NOTES

1. The second author served as the primary trainer.

2. Of the 9 subscales, high scores on all but "staff control" would appear to be consistent with a strengths-based approach. High scores on the staff control dimension reflect a more autocratic environment.

3. More specifically, the hypothesis is that subscale scores on all dimensions except staff control should increase, while the staff control subscale score should decrease.

REFERENCES

Abrams, D. E. (2005). Reforming juvenile delinquency treatment to enhance rehabilitation, personal accountability, and public safety. *Oregon Law Review, 84*, 1001-1092.

Altschuler, D. M., & Armstrong, T. L. (1991). *Intensive community-based aftercare prototype: Policies and procedures.* Baltimore: Johns Hopkins University, Institute for Policy Studies.

Andrews, D. A. (1995). The psychology of criminal conduct and effective treatment. In J. McGuire (Ed.), *What works: Reducing reoffending* (pp. 35-62). New York: John Wiley.

Andrews, D. A., & Bonta, J. (1998). *The psychology of criminal conduct* (2nd ed.). Cincinnati, OH: Anderson.

Andrews, D. A., Zinger, I., Hoge, R. D., Bonta, J., Gendreau, P., & Cullen, F. T. (1990). Does correctional treatment work? A clinically-relevant and psychologically-informed meta-analysis. *Criminology, 28*, 369-404.

Aos, S., Phipps, P., Barnoski, R., & Lieb, R. (2001). *The comparative costs and benefits of programs to reduce crime: Version 4.0.* Olympia, WA: Washington State Institute for Public Policy.

Barnoski, R. (2004). Washington State Juvenile Court Assessment Manual Version 2.1. Olympia: Washington State Institute for Public Policy.

Barton, W. H. (2004). Bridging juvenile justice and positive youth development. In S. F. Hamilton & M. A. Hamilton (Eds.), *The youth development handbook: Coming of age in American communities* (pp. 77-102). Thousand Oaks, CA: Sage Publications.

Barton, W. H. (2006). Incorporating the strengths perspective into intensive juvenile aftercare. *Western Criminology Review, 7*(2), 48-61.

Bazemore, G., & Umbreit, M. S. (1994). *Balanced and restorative justice program summary.* Washington, DC: U. S. Department of Justice, Office of Juvenile Justice and Delinquency Prevention.

Berkowitz, M. W., & Grych, J. H. (1998). Fostering goodness: Teaching parents to facilitate children's moral development. *Journal of Moral Education, 27*(3), 371-391.

Bernard, T. J. (1992). *The cycle of juvenile justice.* New York: Oxford University Press.

Butts, J., Mayer, S., & Cusick, G. R. (2005). Focusing juvenile justice on positive youth development. *Issue Brief # 105.* Chicago: Chapin Hall Center for Children at the University of Chicago.

Cannon, A. (2004, August). Juvenile injustice: Overcrowding, violence, and abuse–state juvenile justice systems are in a shockingly chaotic state. *US News & World Report.* Retrieved August 6, 2004 from: http://www.usnews.com/usnews/issue/040809/usnews/9juvenile.htm.

Clark, M. D. (1997). Strength-based practice: The new paradigm. *Corrections Today, 59*(2), 110-111, 165.

Clark, M. D. (1998). Strength-based practice: The ABC's of working with adolescents who don't want to work with you. *Federal Probation, 62*(1), 46-53.

Cowger, C. D., & Snively, C. A. (2002). Assessing client strengths: Individual, family, and community empowerment. In D. Saleebey (Ed.), *The strengths perspective in social work practice* (3rd ed., pp. 106-123). Boston: Allyn & Bacon.

Deschenes, E. P., & Greenwood, P. W. (1998). Alternative placements for juvenile offenders: Results from the evaluation of the Nokomis Challenge Program. *Journal of
Research in Crime and Delinquency, 35*(3), 267-294.

Franz, J. (1994). Wraparound and the juvenile court: Practical problems in intergalac-
tic communication. Retrieved June 6, 2002 from: http://www.paperboat.com/calli-
ope.juvcourt.html

Franz, J. (2001). Therapeutic jurisprudence. Retrieved June 6, 2002 from: http://
www.paperboat.com/calliope/Thherapeutic.html

Grisso, T., & Barnum, R. (2000). *Massachusetts Youth Screening Instrument-2: User's
manual and technical report.* Worcester MA: University of Massachusetts Medical
School.

Hamilton, S. F., Hamilton, M. A., & Pittman, K. (2004). Principles for youth development. In S. F. Hamilton & M. A. Hamilton (Eds.), *The youth development handbook: Coming of age in American communities* (pp. 3-22). Thousand Oaks, CA:
Sage Publications.

Hawkins, J. D., Catalano, R. F., & Miller, J. Y. (1992). Risk and protective factors for
alcohol and other drug problems in adolescence and early adulthood: Implications
for substance abuse prevention. *Psychological Bulletin, 112*(1), 64-105.

Hawkins, J. D., Herrenkohl, T. I., Farrington, D. P., Brewer, D., Catalano, R. F.,
Harachi, T. W., & Cothern, L. (2000). *Predictors of youth violence.* Juvenile Justice
Bulletin. Washington, DC: U. S. Department of Justice, Office of Juvenile Justice
and Delinquency Prevention.

Heafner, J. (2006a). Transitional services: Training and technical assistance report.
Anchorage, AK: Alaska Division of Juvenile Justice.

Heafner, J. (2006b). Johnson Youth Center: Reentry action plan. Anchorage, AK:
Alaska Division of Juvenile Justice.

Hoge, R., & Andrews, D. (1996). *The Youth Level of Service/Case Management Inventory (YLS/CMI).* Ottawa, Ontario: Carleton University.

Howell, J. C. (2003). *Preventing and reducing juvenile delinquency: A comprehensive
framework.* Thousand Oaks, CA: Sage Publications.

Lerner, S. (1986). *Bodily harm: The pattern of fear and violence at the California
Youth Authority.* Bolinas, CA: Common Knowledge Press.

Lipsey, M. (1992). Juvenile delinquency treatment: a meta-analytic inquiry into the vi-
ability of effects. In T. Cook, D. Cordray, H. Hartman, L. Hedges, R. Light, T.
Louis, & F. Mosteller (Eds.), *Meta-analysis for explanation: A casebook* (pp. 83-127).
New York: Russell Sage Foundation.

Lipsey, M. W., & Derzon, J. H. (1998). Predictors of violent and serious delinquency in
adolescence and early adulthood: A synthesis of longitudinal research. In R. Loeber
& D. P. Farrington (Eds.), *Serious and violent juvenile offenders: Risk factors and
successful interventions* (pp. 86-105). Thousand Oaks, CA: Sage Publications.

Lipsey, M. W., & Wilson, D. B. (1998). Effective intervention for serious juvenile offenders: A synthesis of research. In R. Loeber & D. P. Farrington (Eds.), *Serious and
violent juvenile offenders: Risk factors and successful interventions* (pp. 313-345).
Thousand Oaks, CA: Sage Publications.

Mackin, J. R., Weller, J. M., & Tarte, J. M. (2004). *Strengths-based restorative justice assessment tools for youth: Addressing a critical gap in the juvenile justice system. Final project report.* Portland, OR: NPC Research.
Mackin, J. R., Weller, J. M., Tarte, J. M., & Nissen, L. B. (2005, Spring). Breaking new ground in juvenile justice settings: Assessing for competencies in juvenile offenders. *Juvenile and Family Court Journal,* 25-37.
Maruna, S., & LeBel, T. P. (2003). Welcome home? Examining the "reentry court" concept from a strengths-based perspective. *Western Criminology Review, 4*(2), 1-17.
Mihalic, S., Fagan, A., Irwin, K., Ballard, D., & Elliott, D. (2004). Blueprints for violence prevention. Washington, DC: U. S. Department of Justice, Office of Juvenile Justice and Delinquency Prevention.
Moos, R. H. (1974). *Correctional institutions environment scale manual.* Palo Alto, CA: Consulting Psychologists Press.
Moos, R. H. (1987). *Correctional institutions environment scale: Sampler set.* Palo Alto, CA: Mind Garden.
Nissen, L. B., Mackin, J. R., Weller, J. M., & Tarte, J. M. (2005, Winter). Identifying strengths as fuel for change: A conceptual and theoretical framework for the Youth Competency Assessment. *Juvenile and Family Court Journal,* 1-15.
Northey Jr., W. F., Primer, V., & Christensen, L. (1997). Promoting justice in the delivery of services to juvenile delinquents: The ecosystemic natural wrap-around model. *Child and Adolescent Social Work Journal, 14,* 5-22.
NPC Research. (2006). The Oregon JCP Assessment (2006.1). Portland, OR: [author]. Retrieved March 20, 2007 from: http://www.npcresearch.com/Files/JCP%20screen%202006.1%20_Final%207-06_.pdf
Office of Juvenile Justice and Delinquency Prevention (n.d.). OJJDP Model Program Guide. Washington, DC: U. S. Department of Justice, Office of Juvenile Justice and Delinquency Prevention. Retrieved August 16, 2006 from: http://www.dsgonline.com/mpg2.5/mpg_index.htm
Parent, D. G., Leiter, V., Kennedy, S., Levins, L., Wentworth, D., & Wilcox, S. (1994). *Conditions of confinement: Juvenile detention and corrections facilities. Research summary.* Washington, DC: U. S. Department of Justice, Office of Juvenile Justice and Delinquency Prevention.
Perkins, D. D., Florin, P., Rich, R. R., Wandersman, A., & Chavis, D. M. (1990). Participation and the social and physical environment of residential blocks: Crime and community context. *American Journal of Community Psychology, 18*(1), 83-115.
Pittman, K., & Irby, M. (1996). *Preventing problems or promoting development: Competing priorities or inseparable goals?* Baltimore, MD: International Youth Foundation.
Rapp, C. A. (1998). *The strengths model: Case management with people suffering from severe and persistent mental illness.* New York: Oxford University Press.
Saleebey, D. (Ed.). (2002). *The strengths perspective in social work practice* (3rd ed). Boston: Allyn & Bacon.
Schwartz, R. G. (2001). Juvenile justice and positive youth development. In P. L. Benson & K. Pittman (Eds.), *Trends in youth development: Visions, realities and challenges* (pp. 231-268). Boston: Kluwer Academic Publishers.

Sherman, L., Gottfredson, D., MacKenzie, D., Eck, J., Reuter, P., & Bushway, J. (1997). *Preventing crime: What works, what doesn't, what's promising.* Washington, DC: National Institute of Justice.

Snyder, H. N., & Sickmund, M. (2006). *Juvenile offenders and victims: 2006 national report.* Washington, DC: U. S. Department of Justice, Office of Justice Programs, Office of Juvenile Justice and Delinquency Prevention.

Steinberg, L., Chung, H. L., & Little, M. (2004). Reentry of young offenders from the justice system: A developmental perspective. *Youth Violence and Juvenile Justice, 2*(1), 21-38.

Steinberg, L., & Morris, A. S. (2001). Adolescent development. *Annual Review of Psychology, 52,* 111-139.

Teplin, L. A., Abram, K. M., McClelland, G. M., Dulcan, M. K., & Mericle, A. A. (2002). Psychiatric disorders in youth in juvenile detention. *Archives of General Psychiatry, 59,* 1133-1143.

Torbet, P., & Thomas, D. (2005). *Advancing competency development: A white paper for Pennsylvania.* Pittsburgh, PA: National Center for Juvenile Justice.

Van Wormer, K. (1999). The strengths perspective: A paradigm for correctional counseling. *Federal Probation, 63*(1), 51-58.

Warren, M., Palmer, T., Turner, J., Dorsey, A., McHale, J., Howard, G., Riggs, J., Robberson, J., & Underwood, W. (1966). *Interpersonal maturity level classification: Juvenile diagnosis and treatment of low, middle, and high maturity delinquents.* Sacramento: California Youth Authority.

Wasserman, G. A., Ko, S. J., & McReynolds, L. S. (2004, August). *Assessing the mental health status of youth in juvenile justice settings.* Juvenile Justice Bulletin. Washington, DC: U. S. Department of Justice, Office of Juvenile Justice and Delinquency Prevention.

Appendix A: Youth Competency Assessment (YCA)

[Short Version]

Introduction: It is likely that you will begin the interview by conducting usual Department/Court business: meeting the youth and any other people who are present, introducing yourself, and providing some information about why the youth is there, what they can expect from their visit today and their involvement with you overall, and what expectations the Department/Court has of them. The YCA has the following purposes and goals: (1) To start the process of understanding harm done and how to repair it, (2) To get to know the youth and her/his strengths, and (3) To decide together on competency areas to develop or explore.

Section A: Repairing Harm & Developing Positive Norms and Values

What personal strengths does the youth have that he/she can use to make up for past mistakes?

a. Where have you learned about how to decide right from wrong (e.g., parent, teacher)? What are some examples of what they taught you?

b. Think about what got you in trouble this last time. Who did it hurt? Is there anything you've already done to make up for your actions? What (else) you could do?

c. What could you do to show people that you'll make different decisions in the future? How would these choices benefit you?

Section B: Creating a Healthy Identity

What positive skills and qualities does the youth have that will help her/him succeed? What behaviors does the youth exhibit that reflect a positive identity?
Sample Questions:

d. How do you like to spend your free time?
Hobbies? Sports? Music/Movies? (These questions look for engagement in productive activities)

e. Are you going to school or working anywhere (or have you ever)? What types of things did you enjoy? What were you good at?

f. What types of skills do you have? (This area might need probing and you might need to provide some suggestions)
[Follow up with . . . How do you think these skills will help you in your life?]

g. One of the things we'll be doing together is making some plans for the next few months. What goals would you like to try to achieve in the next _____ (month? 3 months? etc.)? What areas would you like to explore?

h. How would you describe yourself?

i. What is something you like about yourself? (Probe for something more than the superficial)

Section C: Connecting with Family, Peers, and Community

Are there positive people in the youth's life who can serve as a resource for her/him?

j. Who do you spend most of your time with? (Looking for a connection with adults, positive role models)

k. Describe the people you feel most safe with . . . Who are they? If there isn't someone, what are some ways we could help find someone? What is it that makes you feel safe?

l. Who in your life helps you reach your goals or explore your interests? If there isn't someone, what are some ways we could help find someone?

m. Name some people that you respect or that you see doing things you like or appreciate (e.g., teacher, coach, musician, doctor, neighbor). What kinds of things do they do? Who in your family do you admire most? (Why?) Which friend do you admire most? (Why?)

n. Tell me about a time when someone did something nice for you, or helped you out, or gave you something you needed. Why did the person do it?

o. Tell me about a time you did something nice for someone else, or you helped them out, or you gave them something they needed. What types of things do you enjoy doing for others?

p. Who counts on you? [Follow up with . . . What do you do for them?]

> **Note:** If youth is unable to provide positive information about him/herself, it may indicate depression or another underlying issue. Please screen or refer for screening as necessary.

APPENDIX (continued)

YCA Summary and Plan

1. Youth's skills/resources/strengths (can include community or cultural strengths or supports)

   a. _____

   b. _____

   c. _____

2. Short-term competency development/skill building areas:

   a. Mentoring others or being mentored: _____

_____ Review date: _____

   b. Education or Career: _____

_____ Review date: _____

   c. Family or peer relationships: _____

_____ Review date: _____

   d. Repairing harm: _____

_____ Review date: _____

   e. Other: _____

_____ Review date: _____

3. People who can support youth to develop competencies/skills:

   a. Name: _____ Relationship: _____

   b. Name: _____ Relationship: _____

   c. Name: _____ Relationship: _____

4. Summary of youth's long-term goals/plan for future: _____

Now use this information in designing your case plan.

Functional Assessment
in Residential Treatment

W. Guy Tidwell, MA, BCBA

INTRODUCTION

In the latter half of the 20th century, de-institutionalization changed the landscape of residential treatment. Large facilities closed or downsized due to a number of factors including advances in psychology and psychiatry; increased funding for foster care; and decisions by the federal courts regarding the principle of the least restrictive environment (Stein, 1995). As a result, the types of children referred to residential treatment are more challenging; less restrictive alternatives are either not able to provide the needed treatment or unable to safely maintain the placement (Stein, 1995).

Despite the diversity of residential treatment programs in terms of types of children served, sources of funding, size, and regulatory requirements, residential settings have three things in common: (a) twenty four hour care, (b) the goal of discharge to a less restrictive setting, and (c) extensive responsibility for the care and treatment of the children served (Stein, 1995). The broad responsibility and the control of the environment exercised by residential facilities offers a unique advantage to treatment teams faced with the challenge of developing effective interventions for children with behavior disorders. Problem behavior is the product of multiple influences across time and settings (Feldman, 1988; Sturmey, 1996). Residential facilities have access to the child's total environment and therefore have the ability to conduct a thorough assessment of problem behavior.

Behavioral assessment, particularly, functional behavioral assessment (FBA) has distinctive features that match up well with the strengths of the residential facility. First, FBA aims to describe the problem behavior objectively and to identify the environmental factors related to its occurrence (Feldman, 1988; O'Neil, Horner, Sprague, Storey, & Newton, 1997). Residential facilities maintain supervision in all environments and therefore have access to information relevant to assessment. Second, direct observation is central to assessment and FBA uses repeated measures over time (Feldman, 1988; Sturmey, 1996). The use of direct observation over time is problematic because it requires the cooperation of parents, school personnel, etc; this barrier is minimized in residential facilities. Third, the use of interviews is a common feature of FBA (O'Neil et al.); residential facilities have multiple informants readily available across the entire day. Fourth, FBA assumes current variables influence a great deal of problem behavior and that the social context plays a significant role (Carr, Reeve, & Magito-McLaughlin, 1996; O'Neil et al., 1997). In a residential facility, the social context largely involves the staff members. Generally, staff is available for interview, for direct observation by professional staff, and training when needed. Last, the availability of current medical information, health status, medication changes, etc improves the quality of ongoing assessment.

Functional behavioral assessment (FBA), also known as functional assessment, is a process that gathers information about the causes of behavior. Its primary purpose is to identify variables that predict and maintain the occurrence of problem behavior so that effective interventions can be designed (O'Neil et al., 1997). FBA has its roots in operant psychology (Skinner, 1953) and in the field of behavior analysis (Bijou, Peterson, & Ault, 1968). The approach assumes behavior is lawful and purposeful. The context in which behavior occurs defines the meaning of behavior. This context includes the events that precede behavior, known as antecedents, and the events that follow behavior, known as consequences. Together, these antecedent-behavior and behavior-consequence relationships are the contingencies of reinforcement (Skinner, 1953).

FBA has been applied to a wide variety of populations, including special education students, children and adolescents developmental disabilities, children with emotional problems and mental health problems. (Iwatta, Dorsey, Slifer, Bauman, & Richman, 1994; Kern & Dunlap, 1998; Miller, Rathus, & Linehan, 2007; Sturmey, 1996). The types of problems addressed include aggression, self-injury, non-compliance, disruptive behavior, depression, anxiety disorders, delusional behavior, suicidal behavior, and eating disorders. FBA has become standard practice in behavior analysis, recognized and mandated by congress in the public schools (Individuals with disabilities education act, 1997) and recommended for treatment of psychiatric and behavioral problems in mental retardation (Rush & Francis, 2000)

Direct observation by professionals is extremely limited given the 24-hour supervision in residential settings. The contextual variables vary, for example, by shift, location, and the individuals present. In contrast, Para-professional staff, or line staff, is able to observe client problem behavior, and related contextual variables, under naturally occurring conditions. The line staff is in a position to make significant contributions to treatment formulation.

The purpose of this paper is to review two methods of assessment, interviews and narrative A-B-C recording, which involve the participation of line staff. The rationale is that structured interviews can draw out important information about the context in which problem behavior occurs. Second, narrative recording gathers information about problem behavior and its relationship to naturally occurring events. Systematic analysis of this information can identify patterns that otherwise are difficult to detect. In addition, by involving line staff in the assessment process and contributing to treatment formulation, the final product is likely to have a better contextual fit and thus improve the fidelity of implementation (Horner, Sugai, Todd, & Lewis-Palmer, 1999-2000).

BEHAVIORAL PROCESSES MAINTAINING PROBLEM BEHAVIOR

Similar to cognitive psychology (Beck, 1976), the focus of behavior analysis is on current variables that influence behavior. This focus does not ignore temporally distant events, such as early childhood trauma; however, the assumption is that current variables operate to maintain problem behavior. The variables that influence problem behavior are its antecedents and consequences. The goal of FBA is to identify these contextual variables in order to develop effective treatment.

Antecedents

Antecedents are events that precede behavior. There are two categories of antecedents, discriminative stimuli and setting events. A setting event is similar to the concept of an establishing operation (EO). The two concepts are often used interchangeably (e.g., O'Neil et al., 1997), however, this view is not universal (Kennedy & Meyer, 1998). For the purpose of this paper, they are considered functionally the same and term establishing operation or EO is used.

Discriminative Stimuli (Predictors)

Reinforcement of a response in the presence of a stimulus, and not in its absence, makes the response more likely to occur when the stimulus is present. The stimulus that is present during reinforcement is a discriminative stimulus (S^D). A discriminative stimulus or S^D is an antecedent stimulus that predicts the availability of reinforcement for a particular response. An S^D is said to occasion a response, that is, when present it increases the likelihood of a response. In the absence of the S^D, the response is less likely to occur (Michael, 1993). A defining feature of an S^D is its ability to alter the probability of a behavior.

The ring of a phone is an S^D–it predicts that answering the phone will lead to conversation (reinforcement). In the absence of a ringing phone, reinforcement does not follow pick ups. Thus, a phone's ring alters the probability of answering the phone. This example illustrates a sequence of functional relationships: ringing phone (antecedent)–answer phone (behavior)–talk with friend (consequence). Here are two additional examples: (a) A staff member, Mary, often engages a client, Steven, in empathetic, caring conversation when he appears sad, whereas another staff member, Joan, is less likely to engage Steven in conversation. This history results in Mary being discriminative for reinforcement; when Steven feels sad he is more likely to initiate an interaction with Mary; (b) When Bob teases John he gets no reaction. However, when Bob teases Stephen he gets an emotional reaction from Stephen and attention from his peers (laughing). Over time, the presence of Stephen and his peers signal reinforcement for teasing. John and Stephen indicate differential availability of reinforcement for teasing. The presence of Stephen and his peers function as an S^D by altering the probability of teasing.

Discriminative stimuli can turn behavior on and off; however, they do not cause behavior. The causes lie in the consequences. A S^D merely indicates the availability of a consequence.

Establishing Operations (Setting Events)

Consider the previous example of the ringing phone functioning as a discriminative stimulus. When a person is ill and does not want to socialize, talking to others is not a reinforcer. The ringing phone still predicts that answering it will result in a conversation. However, illness has altered the reinforcing value of conversing with others. As a result, the ring tone may not occasion the response of answering the phone. One might say the person is not motivated to talk on the phone. Illness is an example of the second antecedent category, the establishing operation or setting event.

An establishing operation (EO) is an event or operation that has two effects: (1) a momentary change in the reinforcing value of some event, and (2) behavior previously reinforced by that event changes in probability (Michael, 1993). An EO can either increase or decrease the reinforcing value of an event. Water deprivation is an example of an EO. Water deprivation leads to the first effect, it increases the reinforcing value of water (reinforcer-establishing function). This results in the second effect, an increase in behavior previously reinforced by water: buying water, going to the sink, asking for water, etc.

Sleep deprivation is another example of an EO. Loss of sleep might alter the value of a number of activities the next day. Activities that are normally pleasant or tolerable may become aversive events. For example, when sleep deprivation decreases the value of work, it establishes escape and avoidance of work as reinforcement. This change evokes behavior that in the past has avoided work. Sleep deprivation might have multiple effects. Teasing, normally tolerated, may become an aversive event, evoking those behaviors that have terminated teasing in the past.

Illness, pain, nightmares, and changes in medication are all potential EOs. In residential facilities, family visits may function as EOs, particularly when they do not go well. Perceived rejection or abandonment might function to alter the value of attention, increasing the value of empathy, acceptance and reassurance from others. Alternatively, the visit might result in emotional arousal or irritability, making some events such as criticism aversive. Examples EOs in residential facilities include losing privileges such as an outing, family problems, a preferred staff member leaving, breaking up with a girl/boy friend, being victimized or intimidated, missing a meal, doing poorly at school, and sudden changes in routine.

EOs and discriminative stimuli differ in two ways: (1) An EO acts as a motivational variable by altering the potency of a reinforcer. An SD has no effect on reinforcer potency; (2) An SD predicts whether or not reinforcement is available. An EO, in contrast, does not alter or predict the availability of reinforcement. Another difference concerns the temporal relationship to behavior. An S^D occurs immediately prior to a response. EOs, however, can be temporally distant to the behavior, occurring hours or days before.

Problem Behavior

The problem behavior is the behavior targeted for assessment. In order to achieve good reliability between observers, an operational definition is required. The definition should describe the actual actions, intensity, and duration so that different staff members can agree on its occurrence.

Consequences

Consequences maintain a great deal of behavior (Skinner, 1953, 1969). Behavior analysis identifies three types of reinforcing consequences. These are positive reinforcement, negative reinforcement, and automatic reinforcement.

Positive reinforcement. There are two types of positive reinforcement, attention and tangible reinforcement. Attention refers to social consequences provided by another person. Tangible refers to activities and objects that follow a problem behavior. "Positive" refers to consequences that are "added" to the environment after a problem behavior occurs. The problem behavior functions to gain access to these consequences. Attention and tangibles function as reinforcers only when they strengthen a problem behavior.

Negative reinforcement. This term is often confused with punishment. Reinforcement strengthens and increases the frequency of behavior. The use of the word negative refers to the subtraction or removal of an aversive event by a behavior. Negative reinforcement occurs when a behavior terminates, prevents, or delays an aversive event and the behavior becomes more likely to occur for that reason. This process is called negative reinforcement. Negatively reinforced behavior is essentially escape and avoidance behavior or escape motivated behavior. For example, when the radio is too loud (an aversive antecedent event) turning the volume down (behavior), removes the loud music (consequence). Problem behavior that functions to terminate or avoid an aversive event is negatively reinforced.

When staff requests a child to engage in a non-preferred activity (e.g., chores), problem behavior may successfully terminate the staff demands and participation in the chores. In this example, the staff requests are aversive events. Aggression and other disruptive behavior can be very effective in terminating or at least delaying task related demands. Negative reinforcement accounts for both the child and the staff's behavior. The individual's disruptive behavior terminates requests to complete the chores and in addition, negative reinforcement occurs when the staff behavior (discontinuing prompts) ends the client's disruptive behavior (an aversive condition for the staff).

Automatic reinforcement. Socially mediated consequences are not the sole determinant of behavior. Some behavior produces its own reinforcing consequences by either adding stimulation or removing aversive physiological conditions. Research shows repetitive, stereotypic behavior in children with autism is a function of the visual or auditory consequences it produces (Lovass, 1987; Rincover, Cook, Peoples, & Packard, 1979).This is an example of automatic positive reinforcement because the stereotypic behavior adds something to the environment, the visual or kinesthetic stimulation. Automatic negative reinforcement occurs when stereotypic behavior, such as rapid body-rocking or head banging, attenuates or removes an aversive physiological condition such as pain (toothache, headache, etc.).

The Role of Private Events in FBA

Behavior analysis considers thoughts and emotions as behavior (private events) because the verbal community does not have reliable access to them (Skinner, 1953). Thus, private events are amenable to the same type of analysis as overt behavior.

Thoughts and feelings can occur as antecedents, behavior and consequences (Sturmey, 1996). For example, a person diagnosed with obsessive-compulsive disorder might have obsessions (thoughts) about bacteria. The obsessive thoughts are an antecedent to both anxiety and compulsive cleaning. The cleaning results in the removal of the aversive emotional state (consequence). Dougher and Hackbert (2000) provide an example of a person thinking about an upcoming social event. The negative thoughts about his lack of social competence act as an antecedent EO by altering the value of the upcoming party and establishing escape as a reinforcer.

Linehan's dialectical behavior therapy (1993) has been used with success to help individuals with borderline personality disorder and suicidal adolescents (Miller, Rathus, & Linehan, 2007). Functional assessment involves identifying the specific factors contributing to suicidal behavior. The antecedent analysis examines response chains that include thoughts, feelings, overt behavior, and environmental events. Assessment seeks to trace the chain to the environmental variables that occasioned the response chain. The events following suicidal behavior are subjected to a similar analysis to determine the function of the behavior.

Complex Interactions

To summarize, the framework of an FBA includes four elements: an EO, an S^D, the behavior, and its consequence. The four elements usually occur in temporal order as although the EO can occur before the S^D or they can overlap. It is important to recognize that the effects of EOs, S^Ds, and consequences on problem behavior are the result of complex interactions and interdependent relationships.

Problem behavior may have more than one function, that is, more than one type of reinforcement may maintain the behavior. For example, Day, Horner, and O'Neil (1994) conducted experimental functional analyses demonstrating responses with the same topography (self-injury) functioned to escape difficult tasks and to obtain tangible items. These results indicate that self-injury was a member of two response classes, each tied to a different reinforcing outcome. Therefore, a response with dual functions would likely have different antecedent conditions. Self-injury maintained by access to food (tangible) would vary in strength as a function of food deprivation (EO). However, food deprivation would be unlikely to alter the value of escape-motivated behavior. Although the behavior "looks the same," self-injury is functionally two different responses, each with its unique controlling variables. Alternatively, responses with different topographies may serve a similar function. For example, screaming, self-injury and aggression could all be escape motivated. The S^Ds might vary for the different topographies if, e.g., one staff consistently reinforced screaming and another staff consistently reinforced self-injury. Each staff member would predict the same kind of reinforcement but for different response topographies.

As discussed, an EOs have two effects, it alters reinforcer potency and evokes related behavior. However, a third effect occurs when and EO alters reinforcer value the evocative effect of related discriminative also changes. The establishing operation is unique in that it affects all the elements addressed by an FBA-discriminative stimuli, problem behavior, and consequences.

It is increasingly clear that EOs interact with discriminative stimuli and that their combination can exert a strong influence on the occurrence of problem behavior (Carr, Reeve, & Magito-McLaughlin, 1996). Carr et al. (1996) examined the influence of mood (EO) and demands. In the absence of demands, there was no problem behavior; the combination of bad mood plus demands resulted in a problem behavior; and the combination of demands and good mood produced no problem behavior. In a well-controlled study, Horner et al. (1997) demonstrated similar results. Problem behavior occurred almost exclusively during the combination of the EO and S^D. The presentation of the S^D or EO individually resulted in no problem behavior. It appears that neither the EO nor S^D when presented alone is sufficient to evoke problem behavior; however, their combination is a necessary condition. These results support Michael's position that an EO affects consequences and does not act directly on problem behavior. Horner et al. (1997) reported an interesting affect. The EO (cancelled outing) appeared to increase the value of escape motivated behavior and to decrease the value of praise.

Because of these complex interactions, a number of researchers emphasize the need to identify both EOs and discriminative stimuli and to incorporate related strategies in behavioral interventions (Horner et al. 1997; Kennedy & Meyer, 1998).

METHODS OF ASSESSMENT

Goals and Outcomes of FBA

The goals of interviewing and direct observation are to identify the functional relations between problem behavior and its antecedent and consequent events; to design a function based intervention; and, if necessary, to provide information needed to conduct an experimental functional analysis.

Outcomes. The outcomes of FBA are: (a) An operational definition of the target behavior, (b) Identification of the antecedents which predict the occurrence and non-occurrence of problem behavior, (c) Identification of consequences that maintain the problem behavior, (d) generation of hypotheses based on the function(s) of the behavior, (e) development of summary statements which depict the interrelated antecedent-behavior-consequence relationships that support the hypothesis, and (f) development of interventions based on the hypothesized function of the behavior.

There are three general approaches to functional assessment. Indirect assessment, which includes interviews and paper and pencil scales; direct assessment, which involves direct observation in the natural environment; and experimental functional analyses, which manipulate antecedents and consequences using single subject experimental designs.

This paper focuses on the use of interviews and direct observation methods, which can be useful in residential settings.

INDIRECT AND DIRECT ASSESSMENT

Indirect assessment uses rating scales, questionnaires, and interviews. The goal is to obtain information from significant informants such parents, teachers, and staff members (Miltenberger, 1998). This paper only covers interviews because they involve line staff who is able to observe problem behavior under naturally occurring conditions.

Interviews

A number of published interview formats exist (O'Neil et al., 1997; Watson & Steege, 2003). The Functional Assessment Interview Form

(O'Neil et al., 1997) is a comprehensive assessment and has been used in schools for students with problem behavior. The interview assesses antecedents, consequences, and adaptive behavior. The format provides the following information:

1. A clear description of the problem behavior, including rate, intensity, duration, and topography,
2. Potential setting events such as current medications sleep patters, etc.,
3. The immediate antecedents that predict when problem behavior is most likely and least likely to occur (the questions cover the time of day, activities, and people),
4. The types of consequences that follow the problem behavior (for each of the previously identified antecedents the informant identifies what the child "gets" or "avoids"),
5. The efficiency of the problem behavior that includes the immediacy and consistency of reinforcement as well as the effort involved in the problem behavior,
6. Communication skills,
7. Potential positive reinforcers including people, activities, etc.,
8. Information on adaptive behavior that serves the same function as the problem behavior, and
9. Previous interventions used and their effectiveness.

In residential facilities, interviews can provide good information when completed on all shifts. The interview requires 30 to 45 minutes to complete and thus is practical for the busy clinician. However, a novice interviewer is likely to require more time. Conducting the interview with multiple staff members also requires additional time.

Obtaining accurate information from line staff can be complicated. Staff is sometimes reluctant to share information about implementation of current programs by their peers. It is important to establish a non-punitive atmosphere during the interview and make it clear that the goal is to collect information to develop effective treatment. It is important to communicate to line staff that they have valuable information to guide the development of treatment planning. Meeting individually with staff can yield information that staff may not share in a group meeting. When staff do not accurately report how problem behavior was handled, it is difficult to determine how often the problem behavior is reinforced. In my experience, when a group interview yields very little about re-inforcement for a very intense problem behavior, it is useful to assume that reinforcement is occurring and then conduct individual interviews. Intense problem behavior can modify staff behavior causing them to eliminate instructions for therapeutic activities associated with disruptive behavior (Taylor & Carr, 1993).

Narrative A-B-C Recording

The use of A-B-C recording is a useful method for gathering information via direct observation (Horner et al., 1997; Carr et al., 1994). When the interview does not provide sufficient information to develop a hypothesis, direct observation is the next step in assessment. When problem behavior occurs, have the complete a narrative record. The A-B-C format gathers information on immediate antecedents (the A), distant antecedents (EOs), the problem behavior (the B) and consequences (the C). A-B-C recoding is most useful when collected across multiple settings and on at least the day and swing shifts. This is one of the advantages of narrative recording in a residential facility–the ability to collect information about a problem behavior as it occurs under naturally occurring situations across the entire day.

Carr et al. (1994) recommends using index cards for narrative recording. A simple and common format is to divide the card into three sections, one for antecedents, the second for the behavior, and the third for consequences. The dividing lines can run either vertically or horizontally. At the top of the card, provide space for the date and time, the child's name, and the name of the staff that filled out the card. It is important to provide sufficient room for recording. Encourage staff to write on the back of the card if necessary. I have found the cards useful because staff can easily carry them when moving from setting to setting. In addition, the cards can facilitate analysis as described later. Card stock cut in 4"×5.5" provides sufficient room for recording and it fits four cards on an 8"×11" piece of stock to make copies. For staff without experience in narrative recording it is useful to include written prompts on the A-B-C form in each section. For example, in the antecedent section the written prompt might ask, "What interaction occurred just before the problem behavior?" Another common antecedent prompt is to indicate what activity was in progress.

After a week or two of narrative recording, the information may point to a tentative hypothesis; however, potentially important information may appear to be missing. This can be due to inconsistent documentation, which is common. Modification of the form can help capture this information. For example, suppose the morning routine is associated with problem behavior and some records indicate the child woke up in a "bad mood" and is still in bed when the routine begins (potential EO). The team hypothesizes this information could be predictive of problem behavior later in the day. However, some records do not contain this information and it is not clear, if the "bad mood" is occurring infrequently or if some staff are not attending to it. To capture this information, add an additional prompt to the antecedent part of the card to record the presence or absence of the bad mood. A common addition to the A-B-C card is to include client behavior that precedes the problem behavior. These "precursor behaviors" or behavioral antecedents are useful in treatment planning. It can be valuable to prompt the client to engage in coping skills when the pre-cursor behavior occurs. In the consequence section, add prompts, if necessary, to record the effects of staff actions on the child. It is useful to know if the child stops disruptive behavior after a staff interaction.

Staff training is essential when using narrative recording, especially if the staff are new to it. Conduct some direct observations and using the A-B-C format prior to training (Carr et al., 1994). It is not essential that the narratives include instances of the target behavior. A sequence of events, such as a staff member giving an instruction, the client's response, and the actions taken by the staff suffices. Put several examples on a handout for the training. Training is most effective following several guidelines:

1. Use a lecture format to explain the rationale for the narrative recording.
2. Define antecedents, behavior-consequent relationships using the examples on the handouts. You may choose not to use the word antecedent and instead write "before" in the antecedent column. After explaining the A-B-Cs, briefly go over the concept of an establishing operation and give several examples. Ask staff for examples from their experience with different clients. Instruct staff to record setting events and hypotheses on the back of the card, if necessary.
3. Emphasize the importance of recording the social aspects incident (Carr et al., 1994). In most cases, the important information has to do with what the staff say and do preceding the behavior and their response to the problem behavior. Peer interactions just prior to and after the problem behavior are also important. Some staff members do not appreciate the role staff interactions before and after the problem behavior. The tendency is to focus on the client

instead of their interactions. Stress the need for clear records of staff interactions before and after the problem behavior.

4. Explain the need for precise language when describing behavior (O'Neil et al., 1997). Many facilities have jargon that does not adequately convey what the child actually did. Phrases such as destruction of property (DOP) convey little when the narrative does not specify the item or the extent of the damage. If the word "redirect" is part of the vernacular, instruct staff not to use it. If it is used, instruct staff to specify how the client was redirected and to what. It is also beneficial to know what kinds of redirection are effective. Redirection that is verbal vs. hands on is quite different and the latter can be a trigger for problem behavior. Go over words like "angry" and "aggressive" and instruct staff to use specific descriptions of behavior For example, "he hit John hard in the chest with his fist" gives some indication of intensity. A frequently encountered problem is the use of the word "peer" or "client" instead of the names of other clients. There is no confidentiality issue because the narratives are not part of the official record.

5. After the lecture format is completed, provide a handout with a short written vignette describing an interaction with an antecedent, behavior, and consequence. On the same page, include a completed A-B-C record. After reviewing it, hand out blank A-B-C forms and several additional vignettes for practice. Practice is important because it provides a certain level of mastery and fluency that facilitate transfer of learning (Lee & Kahnweiler, 2000). Two or three are sufficient for the first training session. You may decide not to require names but collect the completed samples to help design additional training. After a week or two of narrative recording, schedule a follow up training. Select some completed narratives, several good examples and several that indicate different problems. Type the narratives, leaving out the name of the recorder and use them as a handout. Review the problems revealed by the narratives completed thus far. Providing good examples and poor examples facilitates discriminating what type of information goes in each section. It is important to include the supervisor in all training sessions to provide additional on the floor feedback.

When line staff use A-B-C narratives for the first time, it is beneficial to select the first client carefully. In my experience, staff can view completing narratives as unwanted extra work; initial success can facilitate staff acceptance. Starting with a high frequency problem behavior can quickly generate enough narratives for a good analysis.

O'Neil et al. (1997) recommend that narrative recording continue for about a week with at least a dozen records before analysis begins. However, they work primarily with teachers and parents. In residential facilities, many team members complete the narratives and skill levels are variable. Collecting records for three to four weeks provides better information for two reasons: First, the initial narratives will be quite variable in quality. Second, even after training, 10 to 20% of the narratives will not provide sufficient information. Third, an adequate sampling across settings and time is essential. Two dozen narratives is a minimum target in my experience and more for complex cases.

A-B-C RECORDS:
ANALYSIS AND HYPOTHESIS DEVELOPMENT

After the narratives are collected, the search for patterns begins. Most functional assessment articles lack clear guidelines for analysis of the A-B-C narratives. As Horner (1994) says, "I believe we are better able to describe how to conduct a functional assessment than we are at describing how to use the resulting information to construct a clinical intervention" (p. 403). However, Horner and his colleagues (O'Neil et al., 1997) and Carr et al. (1994) provide practical guidelines for developing hypotheses to drive treatment. Two methods of analysis are given.

Method 1

Review the narratives. Read each card, noting the antecedents and consequences. Write down potential hypotheses on each card. The problem behavior is yelling at and threatening others.

Sort the cards by hypotheses. (Carr et al., 1994). Group the cards by hypotheses using the following categories: (a) Social positive reinforcement (attention), (b) tangible positive reinforcement, (c) escape, and (d) "other." Use the "other" category when the behavior does not seem to have a social function (automatic reinforcement). Place the cards lacking adequate information in a separate area.

Categorize into sub-groups. After sorting the cards in step one, examine each group for patterns. Similar types of antecedents define the patterns. Consider the following hypothetical example. A group of escape related cards results in the following antecedent sub-groups: (a) when requested to complete afternoon chores, (b) when asked to hurry during the morning routine and reminded the bus will arrive soon, (c) when watching TV and asked to help with pre-meal set-up, and (d) when teased by peers.

Staff demands precede the first three categories. Note that the antecedent groups are different. Category b, asked to hurry during a hectic morning routine is quite different from category c, requests to stop watching TV to do meal preparation. The meal set-up shares some features with PM chores-both are task demands. However, the teasing antecedent differs from staff requests. If information indicates that threatening others terminates teasing, then an escape-motivated hypothesis is reasonable. However, peer reinforcement would indicate the threats might be maintained, at least in part, by attention. Additional interviewing, including the client and perhaps peers might help.

When the antecedent sub-categories are complete, some groups may not present a clear picture. When the sub-category is a high frequency or involves a dangerous behavior, additional assessment may be necessary. This may take the form of additional interviews with staff or with the client. At this stage, when presenting to staff it is useful to present the data in an organized fashion, with summary statements and frequencies for the important categories. Staff can often fill in important gaps that can lead to potential interventions. In the hypothetical example, consider that the morning routine, sub-category b, was unclear. If so, completion of specialized A-B-C narratives for several days might be helpful. If some narratives indicated TV watching was a factor in slowing the child's progress in the routine, then additional narratives could track the occurrence and non-occurrence of TV watching every day, whether or not problem behavior occurred. This sort of additional assessment is time limited.

Method 2

An alternative approach is to categorize the cards by antecedent similarity (as opposed to sorting by hypothesized function). Often the antecedent reveals information about the potential function of the behavior. The next step entails examination of each antecedent category for common functions or antecedent sub-categories. This approach can be useful when the consequences are repetitious and similar across most of the narratives. This can occur when the problem behavior is dangerous, thus requiring staff to intervene immediately on each occasion. While this might suggest an attention function, the required intervention by staff may mask other sources of reinforcement. Careful analysis of the antecedent categories can result in alternative hypotheses.

Construct Summary Statements

The next step is to construct summary statements for previously identified antecedent-behavior-consequence relations (O'Neil et al., 1997). This visual aid can help organize and make sense of the analysis completed so far. Below is an example of a hypothetical summary statement.

Distant——Immediate——Problem Behavior——Maintaining			
EO	**Antecedent**		**Consequence**
Unknown	John is asked to do post meal chores	swears at staff and throws objects	other clients get upset; chores not done

A child may have one or several summary statements, depending on the outcome of the narrative sorting completed during the analysis stage.

DESIGNING TREATMENT

The summary statements guide the selection potential interventions. Each of the four elements, EO, immediate antecedent, behavior, and consequence are examined starting with the EO. The objective is to identify potential strategies in each of these areas. Consider the following summary statement.

Distant—(S^D) Immediate—Problem Behavior—Maintaining			
EO	**Antecedent**		**Consequence**
Argument on Phone with Mother the Previous night	asked to start morning routine when in bed	Swears and throws objects at staff	Staff leave and and prompt again in 10 minutes

Establishing Operation

Staff notes that John does not have a real conversation on the phone. He repeatedly asks for things such as movies, candy and visits. When she does not agree, John gets yells at his Mother and she ends the conversation.

When an EO is identified, at least three options are available (Horner, Vaughn, Day, & Ard, 1966): minimize the likelihood the EO will occur, neutralize the effects of the EO, and withhold the S^D. The first option, minimizing the occurrence entails reducing the frequency of phone calls (not an option) or designing an intervention to make the phone calls more positive, thus preventing arguments. The latter has possibilities. The second option, neutralizing the EO involves introducing an event after the EO has occurred (argument with Mother) but before presentation of the S^D. The third option, to withhold the S^D would mean not prompting John to get up the morning following an argument with his Mother; while this has possibilities, the team decides to explore the first two options.

Minimizing the probability of an EO. The team develops the following plan to minimize the likelihood of an argument between John and his Mother. Prior to making a phone call a trusted staff assists John in making a list of the activities John has done the past several days (outings, school projects, etc.) and upcoming fun events. Staff assists John as necessary to write down make notes for reference while on the phone. The team considers role-play sessions with John to teach him how to ask his mother what she has done and how she is doing. If Johns Mother sent him anything, role-playing could include thanking his Mother. The goal is to structure the conversations so they are more positive while at the same time learning some rudimentary conversational skills. The social worker agrees to contact Johns Mother so that she can maximize the discussion around the positive events in the conversation.

Neutralizing the EO. The team explores what positive activities are available that might neutralize after the EO has occurred but before the S^D is presented. The hypothesis is that John becomes hurt and angry when the conversation with his Mother ends in an argument. The result is that the demands of his normal routine become an aversive event and resulting in escape (staying in bed) as a reinforcer. By throwing things at staff, they back off and he remains in bed. The team is able to identify a number of activities that might alter John's emotional state but the timing is a challenge. A neutralizing activity can be presented either before bed or in the morning prior to requests to start his AM routine. The team decides to start with an activity before bed. John enjoys playing cards and the team agrees to start a card game after the phone call before bedtime. As an incentive, they agree to throw in soda and cookies for the players.

Immediate Antecedent

The team decides to approach John differently in the morning. John is asked how he would like staff to wake him up. He responds that he wants to be left alone but agrees that staff can turn on his light. The plan is for staff to remind John three times and to prompt the replacement behavior (see Behavior section).

Behavior

An important goal of the behavior section is the selection of an appropriate response that is functionally equivalent to the target behavior. A functionally equivalent response results in the same consequence as the problem behavior. In this case the consequence is that staff leaves him alone. The goal is for the functionally equivalent response to replace the problem behavior. The rationale supporting the use of a replacement behavior is the concept of a response class. A response class is a group of responses tied to the same reinforcer, in this case, negative reinforcement. All behavior that successfully terminates or delays staff demands and the onset of the AM routine are members of the response class. The member of the response class that John is currently using is throwing things at staff. The members of a response class do not have to be similar responses, that is, they can look quite different from each other. The members of the response class are defined by their common function (escape) and not by their topography. The members of the response class might include rolling over and ignoring staff, swearing, throwing things, and perhaps aggression. Politely asking staff to sleep in 15 more minutes is a potential member of the response class. If the team honors the request, it terminates and delays staff prompting. Thus, a polite request is functionally equivalent to the other members of the response class. If reinforced, it can replace the disruptive behavior. When considering a replacement behavior such as this, the team must decide whether they can honor it. If they cannot, the replacement behavior is not used. However, interventions are planned in the consequence section to compliment the use of the replacement behavior.

Consequences

The team meets with John and explains the use of a replacement behavior. A contract is agreed upon that stipulates: (a) if John uses the replacement behavior, without engaging is disruptive behavior and

(b) if he gets up within 10 minutes of the second prompt, he can earn a special reward. These kinds of interventions are the product of a thorough functional assessment. Each intervention is unique to the identified contextual variables and consistent with John's strengths and interests. It is important to note several characteristics of this intervention. First, it involves skill building, appropriate phone conversation and appropriate ways to terminate staff prompting. Second, it looks at John's quality of life; the use of his conversational skills may improve interactions with his mother and decrease the emotional turmoil it causes. Third, John participated in the development of the treatment. He contributed ideas about how staff might approach him in the morning (turn on his light) and he participated in the development of a contingency contract. The team will collect data on the use of the replacement behavior, the disruptive behavior and his use of improved phone skills. If the intervention does not work as planned, the team will meet again to consider the use of a neutralizing routine.

CASE STUDY

A fifteen-year-old boy, Stephen, engages in self-harm, cutting his legs with sharp objects that he surreptitiously obtains and hides in his room. Lone of sight (LOS) supervision, several room searches per day and occasional body searches are implemented to keep him safe. These measures successfully suppress the cutting behavior, however, but leaving the area, aggression and other disruptive behaviors increase in frequency.

The clinician interviews Stephen and selected staff on all three shifts. A-B-C narrative recording starts immediately on the day and swing shifts. The results indicate multiple influences. Both the interviews and the initial A-B-C records are consistent on at least one series of events: room searches often result in swearing at staff, high arousal, leaving the area, and aggressive behavior when the staff prevents him from leaving the area. This aggression sometimes results in physical restraint. After restraint, he is calmer.

The clinician conducts additional interviews with staff to analyze the chain of events further. Staff indicates several behaviors often occur during the arousal phase that precedes leaving the living area. These include pacing, threats to his peers, statements about hurting himself, and comments that he hates the facility.

In addition, staff report Stephen often argues with staff about rules, about following his program correctly, etc. It appears staff engages Stephen in power struggles; staff are drawn into the arguments about the rules and the veracity of Stephen's statements. During the interview, staff also report that Stephen frequently makes statements that he hates the residential facility and that he will never get to leave and live with his family. The relationship of these events to the problems around room searches is unclear. In an interview with a trusted staff member Stephen reveals staff make him angry when they stare at him and when they mess his room up during room searches. He also reported that when he cut himself he felt calmer.

The team meets and comes to the following hypotheses:

1. Stephens's hopelessness about leaving the facility may act as an EO that increases the aversiveness of the room searches and LOS. There appears to be a relationship between telephone contact and his depressed, irritable mood.
2. Stephen's efforts to engage staff in power struggles increase his arousal levels and may be counter-control measures to "get back" at staff by upsetting them.

The team decides upon a multi-component plan as follows:

1. The team agrees to involve Stephen in his overall treatment planning. A special meeting is held at McDonalds. During the meeting, a long-term goal is established, to live with his family. When asked about short-term objectives to help reach the goal, Stephen identifies cutting and "acting out." The team makes it clear they want to help Stephen reach his goal. Stephen identifies several activities that calm him down and an agreement is reached that staff will prompt him to use his coping skills when pre-cursor behaviors occur. The intent of establishing long term and short-term goals for moving out is to minimize the occurrence of the EO (feeling he will never move out).
2. The team agrees to provide the line staff training to avoid power struggles and how to supervise without staring at Stephen.
3. The team agrees to teach Stephen to make assertive statements when staff stares at his face. Stephen agrees to analogue role-plays and suggests "rewards" for participation. Later the assertive responses are practiced in contrived situations in the living area.

4. The psychiatrist hypothesizes the cutting may function to produce endorphins, endogenous opiates, that may cause his calming and the attenuation of aversive emotional states (automatic reinforcement). The psychiatrist prescribes Naltrexone, a medication that blocks the release of endorphins.
5. The team also agrees to provide Stephen with rewards for tolerating room searches that do not result in disruptive behavior. In addition, the team suggests reinforcement the use of coping responses when prompted by staff.
6. The team agrees to schedule follow up meetings with Stephen on a regular basis.

In this example, the interviews and narrative did not reveal hard evidence of all the relationships but there was sufficient information to develop hypotheses to guide the design of several interventions. Overall, the plan includes measures to minimize the EO, reduce the impact of triggers, to learn valuable coping skills, and to provide reinforcement for participation in the interventions.

CONCLUDING COMMENTS

Residential facilities continue to admit children with very problematic behavior. Functional assessment is an evidence-based practice with strong research supporting its use to understand the determinants of problem behavior and to generate effective treatment (O'Neil et al., 1997). Two methods of assessment, interviews and A-B-C narrative recording match up well with the strengths of residential facilities. Twenty-four hour care provides an opportunity to assess these multiple influences across time and settings. Residential staff is in a unique position to assess the naturally occurring influences on problem behavior and to assist in the development of effective treatment plans. Inclusion of the line staff in the assessment process also increases their sense of participation in the team process. Interventions are more likely to be implemented correctly when the people who implement an intervention assist in its development (Horner et al., 1999-2000).

REFERENCES

Beck, A. T. (1976). *Cognitive therapy and the emotional disorders.* New York: International Universities Press.

Bijou, S. W., Peterson, R. F., & Ault, M. H. (1968). A method to integrate descriptive and experimental field studies at the level of data and empirical concepts. *Journal of Applied Behavior Analysis*, 1, 175-191.

Car, E. G., Levin, L., McConnachie, J. I., Kemp, D. C., & Smith, C. E. (1994). Communication-based interventions for problem behavior: A user's guide for programming positive change. Baltimore, MD: Paul Brookes.

Carr, E. G., Reeve, C. E., & Magito-McLaughlin. (1996). Contextual Influences on problem behavior in people with developmental disabilities. In Koegel, L. K., Koegel, R. L., & Dunlap, G. (Eds.), *Positive behavioral support* (403-423). Baltimore, MD: Paul Brookes.

Day, H. M., Horner, R. H., & O'Neil, R. E. (1994). Multiple functions of problem behaviors: assessment and intervention. *Journal of applied behavior analysis*, 2, 279-289.

Dougher, M. J., & Hackbert, L. (2000). Establishing operations, cognition and emotion. *The behavior analyst*, 23(1), 11-24.

Feldman, R. S. (1988). Behavior Therapy. In Kestenbaum, C. J., & Williams, D. T. (Eds.) *Handbook of clinical assessment of children and adolescents Volume II* (111-1128). NY: New York University Press.

Gardner, W. I. (2002). *Aggression and other disruptive behavioral challenges: Biomedical and psychosocial assessment and treatment*. Kingston, NY: NADD Press.

Hersen, M., & Barlow, D. H. (1976). *Single case experimental designs: Strategies for studying behavior change*. New York: Pergamon.

Horner, R. H. (1994). Functional Assessment: contributions and future directions. *Journal of Applied Behavior Analysis*, 27, 401-404.

Horner, R. H., Vaughn, B. J., Day, M., & Ard, W. R. (1996). The relationship between seting events and problem behavior. In Koegel, L. K., Koegel, R. L., & Dunlap, G. (Eds.), *Positive behavioral support* (381-402). Baltimore, MD: Paul Brookes.

Horner, R. L., Sugai, G., Todd, A. W., & Lewis-Palmer, T. Elements of Behavior Support plans: a technical brief. *Exceptionality*, 8(3), 205-215.

Individuals with Disabilities Education Act. (1997). 20 U.S.C. 1401 et seq.

Iwatta, B. A., Dorsey, M. F., Slifer, K. J., Bauman, K. E., & Richman, G. S. (1994). Toward a functional analysis of self-injury. *Analysis and Intervention in Developmental Disabilities*, 2, 3-20.

Kennedy, C. H., & Meyer, K. A. (1998). Establishing operations and the motivation of challenging behavior. In J. K. Luiselli & M. J. Cameron (Eds.), *Antecedent control* (329-346). Baltimore, MD: Paul H. Brookes.

Kobe, F. H., & Mulick, J. A. (1995). Mental retardation. In R. T. Ammerman & M. Hersen (Eds.), *Handbook of Child Behavior therapy in the psychiatric setting* (pp. 153-180). New York: Wiley-Interscience.

Lee, C. D., & Kahnweiler, W. M. (2000). The effect of a mastery learning technique of the performance of a transfer of training task. *Performance Improvement Quarterly*, 13(3), 125-139.

Linehan, M. M. (1993). Cognitive-behavioral treatment of borderline personality disorder. New York: Guilford Press.

Lovass, I., Newsom, C., & Hickman, C. (1987). Self-stimulatory behavior and perceptual reinforcement. *Journal of Applied Behavior Analysis*, 20, 45-68.

Michael, J. (1993). Establishing operations. *The behavior analyst*, 16, 191-206.

Miller, A. L., Rathus, J. H., & Linehan, M. M. (2007). *Dialectical behavior therapy with adolescents*. New York, NY: Guilford Press.

Miltenberger, R. G. (1998). Methods for assessing antecedent influences on challenging behavior. In J. K. Luiselli & M. J. Cameron (Eds.), *Antecedent control* (pp. 47-66). Baltimore, MD: Paul Brookes.

O'Neil, R. E., Horner R. H., Albin, R. W., Sprague, J. R., Storey, K., & Newton F. S. (1997). *Functional Analysis and program development for problem behavior: A practical handbook (2nd ed.)*. Pacific Grove, CA: Brooks/Cole.

Reiss, S., & Aman, M. G. (Eds.) (1998). *Psychotropic medications and development disabilities. The international consensus handbook*. Columbus: Ohio State University, Nisonger Center.

Repp, A. C., & Horner, R. H. (1998). *Functional analysis of problem behavior: From effective assessment to effective support*. Belmont, CA: Wadsworth.

Rincover, A., Cook, R., Peoples, A., & Packard, C. (1979). Sensory extinction and sensory reinforcement principles for programming multiple adaptive behavior change. *Journal of Applied Behavior Analysis*, 12, 221-233.

Rush, A. J., & Frances, A. (2000). Expert consensus guideline series. Treatment of psychiatric and behavioral problems in mental retardation. [Special issue]. *American Journal of Mental Retardation*, 105(3).

Sidman, M. (1960). *Tactics of scientific research*. New York: Basic Books, Inc.

Skinner, B. F. (1953). *Science and human behavior*. New York: Free Press.

Skinner, B. F. (1969). *Contingencies of reinforcement: A theoretical analysis*. New York: Appleton-Century-Crofts.

Stein, J. A. (1995). *Residential treatment of adolescents & children*. Chicago: Nelson-Hall.

Sturmey, P. (1996). *Functional analysis in clinical psychology*. Chichester, UK: Wiley.

Taylor, J. C., & Carr, E. G. (1993). Reciprocal social influences in the analysis and intervention of severe challenging behavior. In Reichle, J. R., & Wacker, D. P. (Eds.), *Communicative alternatives to challenging behavior* (pp. 63-82). Baltimore, MD: Paul Brookes.

Watson, T. E., & Steege, M. W. (2003). *Conducting school-based functional assessments*. New York: Guilford Press.

The Assessment of Staff Satisfaction as Compared to Client Satisfaction in Two Department of Social Service Residential Treatment Facilities

Amy Levin, PhD
James T. Decker, PhD, LCSW

INTRODUCTION

Burnout, after a period of time, produces distrust, negativism, and inflexibility, which ultimately isolates childcare workers from helping their residents in a personal way (Decker, Bailey & Westergaad, 2002). A discussion of the causes and effects of burnout is necessary when examining levels of staff satisfaction and how it relates to client satisfaction, especially in the residential treatment field where workers face high levels of stress on a day-to-day basis. It is estimated that the turnover rate of childcare workers in residential treatment facilities is 26 to 41 percent each year (Curry, McCarragher, & Dellmann-Jenkins, 2005; Whitebook, Philips, & Howes, 1989) (Also see Dietzel & Coursey, 1998; Manlove & Guzell, 1997; Onyett, Pillinger, & Muijen, 1997; Ross, 1983; Whitaker, 1996).

Burnout is a key word frequently used in the field of social work and human services in general. Burnout is defined as a breakdown of the psychological defense that workers use to adapt to and cope with intense job related stressors and a syndrome in which a worker feels emotionally exhausted or fatigued, withdraws emotionally from their clients, and perceives a diminution of their achievements or accomplishments (Kreisher, 2002). There are many different symptoms of burnout, including recurrent bouts of the flu, gastrointestinal problems, headaches, fatigue, insomnia, substance abuse, poor self esteem, withdrawal behavior, difficulty in interpersonal relationships, rigid adherence to rules, inability to concentrate, and intolerance towards and tendency to blame clients for their own problems (Arches, 1985). One factor rated by staff as a significant source of stress is the challenging behavior (e.g., self-injury, aggression, destructive behavior) of clients (Rose, Home, Rose, & Hastings, 2004). There is also direct evidence suggesting that staff who are exposed to more frequent, and more challenging behaviors are at increased risk of stress, burnout, and mental health problems (Rose, Home, Rose, & Hastings, 2004).

When a worker can no longer tolerate occupational pressures and feels completely overwhelmed by stress, he is likely to reach a breaking point and experience burnout, which may change attitudes and behavior. Workers in residential settings, especially workers who have extensive interaction with demanding sub-populations, are more vulnerable to high degrees of burnout (Decker et al., 2002; Weisberg, 1994). Many causes of burnout for residential child care workers include: long hours, emotional strain, working off hours such as overnight shifts, financial strain, large amounts of paperwork, large caseloads, lack of supervision, and lack of training (Decker et al., 2002).

Job satisfaction has been found to be a strong and consistent predictor of intention to leave as well as turnover (Agho, Mueller, & Price, 1993; Blankertz & Robinson, 1997; Hillman, 1997; Ito, Eisen, Sederer, Yamada, & Tachimori, 2001; Lum, Kervin, Clark, Reid, & Sirola, 1998; Manlove & Guzell, 1997; Tett & Meyer, 1993). Research on job satisfaction clearly shows that lack of resources, less rewarding work conditions, lack of support from supervisors and coworkers, and heavy workloads all produce dissatisfied employees (Mueller & Wallace, 1996; Tyler & Cushway, 1998).

Organizational commitment, a work attitude generally referring to the strength of an employee's identification with and involvement in the organization, is a strong predictor of intent to stay among residential child care workers (Landsman, 2001; Mor Barak, Levin and Nissly, 2001) as well as employees in other fields (Lum et al., 1998; Tett & Meyer, 1993).

Well-being has consistently been shown to influence both job satisfaction (Koeske & Kirk, 1995; Siu, Cooper, & Donald, 1997) and organizational commitment (Weaver, 2002). Finally, a review of the literature yields strong evidence for an association between job satisfaction and organizational commitment (Jayaratne, 1993; Knoop, 1995; Koeske & Kirk, 1995; Testa, 2001; Tett & Meyer, 1993), but it is not clear whether satisfaction is a precursor to commitment or whether commitment influences one's level of satisfaction (Mor Barak, Levin, Nissly, & Lane, 2005).

There are many issues that are the result of employee burnout, especially in non-profit residential organizations. In many agencies, *employee turnover* rate is the number one issue for Human Resources. Several studies have linked burnout to employee turnover or intention to leave (Ellett, 2004; Garland, 2002; Smith, 2005). A high turnover rate often will interrupt client care and can cause a higher burnout rate for the employees still working in the facility. An interruption of client care can be detrimental and can cause a lower client satisfaction rate. Labor turnover is an inevitable phenomenon in an organization's life cycle that involves redundant monetary and non-monetary costs, particularly when efficient and experienced workers, with substantial amounts of investments in their human capital (schooling, experience, skills), leave voluntarily. Because of this, management is oftentimes preoccupied with a constant search to identify signals of potential labor turnover (Weisberg, 1994). Thus, this study asks the following questions: Does the level of job satisfaction affect the quality of care the client is receiving? How can agencies provide better care for their staff in order to provide care for their clients? Can burnout be prevented?

METHODOLOGY AND SAMPLING

This exploratory study looked at the rate of staff satisfaction as compared to client satisfaction. This study employed a cross-sectional analysis of staff and clients self-report on overall level of satisfaction. The authors looked at whether or not the level of staff satisfaction is equal to the level of client satisfaction in two residential treatment programs for children in care of the Department of Social Services (DSS) in the state of Massachusetts (one treatment center was all young women and the other treatment center was all young men). Day treatment staff consisted of sixteen staff members (eight males and eight females), eight staff members from each organization were interviewed as was thirty-one clients; sixteen female clients were from one organization and fifteen males were from a second organization. The age range for staff was 22 to 41 and the age of clients ranged from 6 to 14.

A graduate student finishing her research project received approval from the college institutional review board and obtained permission from the Department of Social Services, Fall River Area Office, to speak with both staff and clients (children). An interview was conducted with each day treatment staff person at both residential treatment center, and all clients were interviewed as well. Prior to the interview, each staff and client was provided with a consent form. For the clients, the consent form was also explained to them. Demographic data was obtained from each staff member and client. For the staff, there were 20 questions, of which nine were scaled and the rest were open ended. The clients were asked 26 client satisfaction questions of which fifteen were scaled and the rest open ended. The questions asked were to assess level of satisfaction and burnout among the employees in a residential treatment facility.

Four items relating to what staff liked best about their job yielded responses on a 5-point Likert scale from *not at all* to *a lot.* Item responses were summed. Scores ranged from 0 to 16. In Table 1 it is apparent that there are lower mean scores (8.8 to 11.2) while the only score to receive a mean of 16 was with "working with kids." The lower mean scores for flexibility and freedom suggest higher levels of job-dissatisfaction that can lead to burnout. Five other items for the staff looked at what they like least about their job, and also yielded responses on a five-point Likert scale from *strongly disagree to strongly agree.* Item responses are summed then averaged with scores ranging from 0 to 20. The mean range was from 10.4 to 15.4 (out of a possible 20) with higher means suggesting a greater perceived potential for burnout. Staff members appear to feel most dissatisfied with their salary, client related issues and with the hours that they must work. There were eleven open-ended questions that were used to develop greater insight into issues of burnout, job satisfaction, organizational commitment and well-being for staff. See appendix for a copy of the items in the survey.

Eight items for the clients addressed what goals they felt that they accomplished during residential care, and yielded responses on a 5-point Likert scale from *not at all* to *a lot.* Item responses are summed then averaged. Total scores ranged from 0 to 32, with higher scores suggesting greater goal accomplishment. The current sample had mean scores ranging from 21 to 28, signifying that overall clients felt that they had accomplished several of the goals of the program. Of the seven scaled

TABLE 1. Education and Experience Within Age Categories N = 16

Age	Education		Years in Human Services	Sex	Staff N =16
22-28	31.25% (n = 5)	BA or BS Degree	0-2	Female	N = 3
				Male	N = 2
	12.5% (n = 2)	Some College		Female	N = 1
				Male	N = 1
29-38	50% (n = 8)	Some College	3-5	Female	N = 2
				Male	N = 4
	12.5% (n = 2)	Graduate Degree			
				Female	N = 1
				Male	N = 1
39 and above	6.25% (n = 1)	High School	7 Plus Years	Female	N = 1

questions related to "client's feelings and thoughts on residential care," scores ranged from 0 to 28, with higher scores suggesting greater satisfaction. The current sample had mean scores ranging from 21 to 28, indicating that overall they were highly satisfied with their residential care experiences. There were eleven open-ended questions that were used to assess level of client satisfaction. It was the authors hope that these questions would develop greater insight into perception of services being received.

RESIDENTIAL STAFF

Data was collected from a questionnaire completed by each member of the staff. Demography data is listed in table one, which looks at age, level of education and amount of time employed in the human service field. Staff education and experience levels are described across three age categories: 22-28, 29-38, and 39 and above. Of the staff that ranged in age from 22-28, five have their BA/BS degree (three women and two men) and two have some college (one women and one male) and all seven have up to two years experience in the human service field. For the age group between 29 and 38, two women and four male staff members have some college and one women and one male staff member have graduate degrees and have worked in the human service field between three and five years. The only staff in the 39 and above age category is a woman who has been employed at the residential treatment facility the longest. She has a high school degree with over seven years of experience.Previous studies (Curry, McCarragher, & Dellmann-Jenkins, 2005; Decker, 2002) have demonstrated a relationship between age with job satisfaction and burnout; younger workers express more job dissatisfaction than older workers. Age is also strongly correlated with childcare workers feeling a lack of supervision (Decker, 2000). In this present study, looking at educational backgrounds of workers who had either a BA or MA degree, we found that their level of job satisfaction and burnout was greater than those who had less than a college degree. When looking at organizational commitment for staff, we found that workers with educational levels of at least a BA degree were more likely to feel job dissatisfaction than those workers who have less education. We also found that a relationship exists between tenure with the organization and job satisfaction and burnout; employees who have been with an organization for a longer period of time are more satisfied, but also suffer from greater levels of burnout. Well-being has consistently been shown to influence both job satisfaction (Koeske & Kirk, 1995; Siu, Cooper, & Donald, 1997) and organizational commitment (Weaver, 2002). Regardless of age, education, gender, or years of experience, all employees in the current study felt inadequate pay was a major issue in relation to job satisfaction and levels of burnout.

If we look at Table 2 we can see that all of the employees stated that one of the things they liked best about their jobs was working with children. Utilizing standardized open-ended questions related to what else staff liked about their job, seven staff wrote "Seeing the progress that some clients make," "interactions with clients on a personal basis," "being a role model," "knowing that they are really good kids," "when a child is able to go home to his family," "talking with other staff about their ideas on how work with some of the more troubling kids," and "making a difference in children's lives" as a few of the things they liked best about their jobs.

Staff felt that "management flexibility around scheduling" and "flexibility in overtime hours" was positive. Another example of flexibility on the job came from a staff member who wrote "I am not in a cubicle in front of a computer all day; I enjoy being able to move freely and do a variety of different things with the clients throughout the course of the day," which supports job satisfaction (Koeske & Kirk, 1995; Siu, Cooper, & Donald, 1997) and organizational commitment (Weaver, 2002).

Table 3 looks at what staff like least about their jobs.

Open-ended questions provided additional information related to what staff liked least about their jobs. Issues that staff felt strongly about that had a negative effect on their work were: "putting children in restraints"; "hours that they worked"; "turn-around shifts"; "being on call"; and "working evenings and weekends." They also felt that the frequent

TABLE 2. What Do You Like Best About Your Job? N = 16

Questions	Not at all	A little	Somewhat	Quite a bit	A lot	Mean
Working with kids					100% (n=16)	16
Team work		25% (n=4)	25% (n=4)	25% (n=4)	25% (n=4)	11.2
Flexibility	12.25% (n=2)	25% (n=4)	31.25% (n=5)		31.25% (n=5)	10
Freedom	31.25% (n=5)	25.% (n=4)	12.25% (n=2)		31.25% (n=5)	8.8

TABLE 3. What Do You Like Least About Job? N = 16

Questions	Strongly disagree	A little	Somewhat	Agree	Strongly agree	Mean
Salary				50% (n=8)	50% (n=8)	15.4
Client related issues		12.5% (n=2)		50% (n=8)	37.5% (n=6)	13.2
Hours			12.5% (n=2)	62.5% (n=10)	25% (n=4)	13.2
Performing restraints on the children			31.25% (n=5)	50% (n=8)	18.75% (n=3)	12.4
Frequent turnover and lack of staff	12.5% (n=2)	25.% (n=4)	25% (n=4)	25% (n=4)	12.5% (n=2)	10.4

"turn-over of staff" and "lack of sufficient staff" was another thing they liked least about their positions. "Salary" was a major issue for all of the participants. Client related issue was also talked about, which included "being spit on," "not as many activities to take children on," "not being able to express their judgment where kids are being place upon discharge," and "extremely difficult kids." These findings are consistent with what other research studies on job satisfaction demonstrates: that lack of resources, less rewarding work conditions, lack of support from supervisors and coworkers, and heavy workloads all produce dissatisfied employees (Mueller & Wallace, 1996; Tyler & Cushway, 1998).

Other standardized open-ended questions related to childcare workers satisfaction with their positions yielded the following responses: When asked what would make your job more satisfying, "all" stated that more money would make the position much more satisfying. They went on to state that other conditions would improve their level of satisfaction, such as: "better hours," "more respect from management," "more responsibilities and clinical time with the children," "having management be on the floor more often," and "being able to give the children more one-on-one time."

On the other hand, we wanted to know if in fact they felt positive towards management and we asked if management is attentive to their needs, and most said yes. When looking at the working environment and whether or not the program encourages teamwork, seven stated always, while nine said rarely or sometimes. When asked if they felt like their work was valued and appreciated by management, one half said sometimes and the other half said always. While addressing issues of monetary compensation and other perks of the job, only six staff responded positively; others stated: "when I talk to other workers outside of this program, I am embarrassed when I learn of their salaries and benefits." "I knew I was under paid, but not this much, based on the time I spend here." "I love working with the kids, but I also have to pay the bills." "Based on the pay, it does not surprise me that we have so much turn over and that is too bad since most of the staff are really committed to the children." Staff were split 50-50 on whether or not the organization encouraged professional development. Interestingly, when asked if they felt satisfied with their jobs, 81.25% said always. Research on organizational commitment, a work attitude generally referring to the strength of an employee's identification with and involvement in the organization, is a strong predictor of intent to stay among residential child care workers (Landsman, 2001; Mor Barak, Levin, & Nissly, 2001).

RESIDENTIAL CLIENTS

Data related to client satisfaction was collected from a standardized discharge questionnaire when clients were ready to leave the residential treatment facility. Data was collected from 31 clients ranging in age from six to fourteen. Table 4 breaks down the clients by age and gender. Based on the age of the clients, questions were developed that the researchers felt were age appropriate. Clients were not coached on interpreting what was meant by each question.

When clients were asked which of the eight program goals (see Table 5 below) they accomplished while in care, four of the 6-8 year olds stated that being honest was a primary goal achieved during their residential treatment; one felt being a kid was a goal and two stated that they needed to follow the rules. For the 9-11 year olds, four felt their primary goal was to be respectful, three felt it was important to learn how to express themselves appropriately, one stated that being a kid was important, one felt a goal was learning to focus on themselves, one felt is was

TABLE 4. Gender of Clients by Age Categories N = 31

Age	Female N=16	Male N=15
6-8	3	4
9-11	5	6
12-14	8	5

TABLE 5. Goals Accomplished by Clients During Residential Care N = 31

Questions	Strongly disagree	A little	Somewhat	Agree	Strongly agree	Mean
Learn to follow the house rules				25.79% (n=8)	74.2% (n=23)	29.4
Be respectful			16.13% (N=5)	41.95% (N=13)	41.95% (n=13)	26.4
Focus on yourself	3.22% (n=1)	32.27% (n=10)		32.27% (n=10)	32.27% (n=10)	22.2
Be honest		12.9% (n=4)	32.27% (n=10)	41.95% (N=13)	12.9% (n=4)	22
Express yourself appropriately		32.27% (n=10)	29.03% (n=9)	19.35% (n=6)	19.35% (n=6)	20.2
Speak up for yourself	25.79% (n=8)	32.27% (n=10)	16.13% (n=5)		25.79% (n=8)	16.6
Be a kid	60.06% (n=18)	60.06 % (n=18)	9.67% (n=3)		6.45% (n=2)	14.6
Listen for the first time	60.06% (n=18)	30.03% (n=9)	6.45% (n=2)		6.45% (n=2)	10.04

important to listen and one felt is was important to follow the house rules. Three of the 12-14 year olds stated that being respectful was a goal for them, one stated learning to express herself was a goal, three felt speaking up for themselves was important, two expressed a need to focus on themselves, one stated she needs to learn how to listen and two stated it was important to follow the rules. Other goals to be accomplished included controlling anger, being proud of themselves and staying positive.

The following standardized open-ended questions highlight the qualitative replies of the respondents: How do you feel about leaving the program? Most stated they were happy to be leaving; "I feel happy because I get to go back home today." On the other hand, clients stated that they had mixed emotions about leaving; "I don't really want to leave because I have a lot of friends here, but I still am happy that I am going to a new place." One client was confused and stated "Well I feel okay because I get to move on . . . I get a step up on going home even though I am going to another group home. . . . but I feel bad that I have to leave wonderful people at the program." Still other clients stated that they felt scared or sad because they were leaving the program; "I am kind of worried about what is going to happen next," "I hate it that I have to leave and go to another group home." Another client stated that he did not know how he felt about leaving.

When we asked clients what staff could do better or differently, nine said "they didn't know or nothing," two clients said "have no rules or different rules," five clients stated "they should have better or different activities," "let us play video games," "take us for a walk." Three clients stated that the staff could be nicer, "don't yell as much." One client stated that the staff could let them talk to their families; "let me talk to my dad."

Looking at Table 6 we asked clients if they felt that their needs were met at this residence.

TABLE 6. Clients Feelings and Thoughts on Residential Care N = 31

Questions	Not at All	A Little	Somewhat	Quite a bit	A Lot	Mean
Do you think the staff at this residence respected you?	0	6.4% (n=2)	6.4% (n=2)	16.1% (n=5)	71% (n=22)	28
Did you respect the program?	6.4% (n=2)	3.2% (n=1)	6.4% (n=2)	19.4% (n=6)	58.7% (n=18)	24.8
Do you feel that your needs were met at this residence?	3.2% (n=1)	12.8% (n=4)	22.6% (n=7)	19.4% (n=6)	41.9% (n=13)	23.8
Do you think you will be able to make better choices in the future because of the work you did here?	12.9% (n=4)	3.2% (n=1)	6.4% (n=2)	22.6% (n=7)	54.8% (n=17)	23.6
Do you think you have learned to get along better with others?	6.4% (n=2)	16.1% (n=5)	3.2% (n=1)	22.6% (n=7)	51.6% (n=16)	23.2
Has the program helped you and your family get along better?	9.7% (n=3)	20% (n=9)	3.2% (n=1)	19.4% (n=6)	38.7% (n=12)	21.6
Do you think the program staff helped you understand yourself better?	22.6% (n=7)	12.9% (n=4)	3.2% (n=1)	25.8% (n=8)	35.5% (n=11)	21

DISCUSSION

Of the 31 clients involved in receiving services at two different residential treatment centers, 69% of those clients expressed overall satisfaction. Eighty-seven percent felt respected by the staff and 78% stated that they respected the program. On the other hand only 58% felt that this program was positive in its goal of the family reunification process.

To date, there is very little research related to young children as clients and their level of satisfaction with the services they receive. We set out to explore whether or not there is a relationship between staff level of satisfaction and client satisfaction with services.

Clearly, this study needs to be replicated in order to show a connection between residential childcare workers level of satisfaction and client satisfaction. More importantly, replication of this study needs to take place with larger samples from a greater variety of backgrounds. Small samples generally do not provide enough power, when traditional data analytic techniques are used, to be able to detect meaningful differences, and do not allow the researcher enough flexibility to exam the information in all its complexity (Decker et al., 2002). Investigating residential childcare worker's adjustment by age, education, gender and type of experience is difficult unless the sample is quite large. Alternatives to the large data set also need to be considered. For example, the richness of information obtained is preserved when using qualitative methodologies such as interviewing, and smaller samples are appropriate for these types of investigations (Decker et al., 2002). It is for these reasons that the current study is exploratory in nature. Even with the small sample size, the results of this study can begin to explore its contribution to theory.

Looking at *young children as clients and their satisfaction* with the services they received at two different residential treatment centers (one for young girls and one for young boys), the concept of *alienation* could be used to explain their reactions to our questions. It is a useful concept since it deals with the interplay between an individual and the institutions of his/her society. According to Seeman (1959), there are four key elements in acquiring a legitimate identity within a social order: (1) A sense of competence; (2) A sense of usefulness; (3) A sense of belongingness; and (4) A sense of power or potency (pp. 786-787). The common theme of these four elements is their institutional character. In the present study, 87% of the clients expressed that staff respected them, which demonstrates that they are acquiring a positive sense of identity through "a sense of competence, usefulness and belongingness." Looking at acquiring a sense of "power," 78% stated that they developed a respect for the program, and 77% stated they will be able to make better choices in the future. Future studies should be designed to explore alienation in relation to satisfaction with services received.

By examining the availability of opportunities for young children to gain access to feelings of competency, usefulness, belongingness, and power through active roles in residential treatment institutions, we can seek to understand the process of young children in a treatment community. We can explore both their pleasures and their frustrations. From this understanding, we can begin the process of grounding a theoretical understanding of young children and client satisfaction.

PRESENTATION OF DATA-STAFF

Although there may be a dearth of hard demographic literature, there is a great deal of literature that focuses on the causal factors of residential childcare workers on *burnout* and *job satisfaction*. There are several recurring themes in this study about causal factors related to *burnout*.

Emotional exhaustion creates emotional perceptions. The parts of their job that the workers in this study did not care for were putting children in restraints, the number of hours that staff had to work, and then have turn around shifts along with working evenings, turnover of staff, money issues, being treated disrespectfully, and not being involved in placement decision at discharge, to name a few examples, only reinforces what Kreisher (2002) defines as burnout. This burnout is a breakdown of the psychological defense that workers use to adapt to and cope with intense job related stressors and a syndrome in which a worker feels emotionally exhausted or fatigued, withdraws emotionally from their clients, and perceives a diminution of their achievements or accomplishments. Although the workers in the current study did not show major signs of burnout, there were several tasks related to their jobs that they did not enjoy performing. Over time, continuing to have to perform these tasks may lead these workers to experience greater levels of burnout. For this study, it is important to point out that seven of the sixteen employees had two years or less experience as child care workers.

There are several recurring themes about causal factors related to *job satisfaction*. The literature speculates that more money, more responsibilities and more one on one time with clients would make the position more satisfying (Mueller & Wallace, 1996; Tyler & Cushway, 1998). It

is also important for management to be more visible and more appreciative of the difficult work that staff members do, and more encouraging
of professional development (Decker et al., 2002). Finally, job satisfaction is related to level of team work, the more employees work together,
the more satisfied they will be with their job. Research on job satisfaction
clearly shows that lack of resources, less rewarding work conditions,
lack of support from supervisors and coworkers, and heavy workloads
all produce dissatisfied employees (Mueller & Wallace, 1996; Tyler &
Cushway, 1998).

The staff in this sample is very content regarding the work that they
do with the children in the residential treatment facility. All 16 staff
members surveyed love working with their clients. Over thirty percent
enjoy the flexibility and freedom that come with the job; however, only
twenty five percent feel that they work as a team with their colleagues.
In terms of their dislikes related to the job, fifty percent feel that they are
not properly compensated for the difficult work that they do. Thirty
eight percent feel that there are multiple client related issues that add to
their dissatisfaction, and twenty five percent do not care for the hours
that they must work. Despite the fact that this group of workers are quite
satisfied with the work that they do, there are still several areas that
those sampled feel could be improved in order to increase level of job
satisfaction.

PRESENTATION OF DATA-CLIENT

Based on the staff's program goals for the 31 clients, twenty three
percent met the goal of being respectful and only nineteen percent met
the goal of expressing themselves appropriately. There is a major dis-
connect between what the programs goals are in terms of changes
sought for the client's behavior and self reported changes in client behavior. However, clients did note that their goals, which were controlling anger, being proud of themselves (self-esteem) and staying positive
(self-esteem) were different from the program goals.

In terms of the therapeutic value related to residential care for young
people, 61% felt that their needs were met quite a bit or a lot; they also
felt that the staff respected them, as 87% stated that they felt respected
either quite a bit or a lot. Fifty eight percent of participants felt the program helped them and their families; however, only half the clients felt
that staff helped them gain better insight into themselves.

In the data presented, only four clients felt it important to "be honest"; only 41% felt that "being respectful" was important; and only eight clients felt that they could "speak up for themselves." Only two felt like they could "be a kid"; 32% felt like they "focus on themselves." Twenty six percent of the clients are either "sad or scared" of leaving the program and another 26% "have mixed emotions" about leaving, which demonstrates that little insight was provided into issues related to the children and their families.

CONCLUSIONS

Satisfied employees tend to be more creative and committed to their employers, and recent studies have shown a direct correlation between staff satisfaction and client satisfaction (Landsman, 2001; Syptak, Marsland, & Ulmer, 1999). Kaldenberg and Regrut (1999) state that customer or client satisfaction largely depends on employees who deliver services to the customer or client. Profits result from the positive relations between organizational structure, employee satisfaction and customer satisfaction (Kaldenberg & Regrut, 1999). As a result of happier employees, the clients' needs are met. When a client is satisfied, employees will feel a sense of accomplishment and are more likely to be satisfied with their jobs. If employees are dissatisfied, they are more likely to provide poor services, which in turn may lead to client dissatisfaction. On the other hand, if employees are committed and satisfied, they are more likely to provide excellent services, which should result in client satisfaction.

This study demonstrates that in two residential facilities, the majority of both staff and clients were satisfied. When asked directly if staff were satisfied with their jobs, 100% stated they were on some level–13 stated always and 3 noted sometimes. Although clients were never directly asked if they were satisfied during their stay at the residential facilities, based on their responses to the questions outlined in Tables 5 and 6 concerning what staff could do differently, and clients thought and feelings about the help they received from staff while in care, it appears that they were quite satisfied overall. We feel that the instrument used to assess level of satisfaction and burnout among the workers can be used in other residential treatment facilities in order for those organizations to measure their staffs level of commitment to the organization, as well as ways in which to improve overall satisfaction and reduce employee burnout.

Understandably, working in a residential facility is not easy, nor is being locked up in a facility away from family and friends. There are many factors that relate to staff not being satisfied with their jobs. There are problems with staff not feeling adequately compensated for their work and feeling as if they are not given proper supervision. Staff also feel unappreciated, and that they lack sufficient training for the work that they must do. There is a sense of a lack of opportunities for professional growth, and lack of teamwork among colleagues. It is well known that a satisfied staff provides better care for residents, which in turn creates a more satisfied client; therefore, what can be done to improve employee level of job satisfaction?

Limitations

There are several limitations to the current study. First of all, due to the nature of an exploratory study, the sample size is extremely small, which reduces the possibility of generalizability. We also did not look at any other institutions as a comparison group for both staff and clients. Replications of this study should include larger sample sizes as well as comparison groups to accuracy of the results and future generalizability.

SUGGESTIONS FOR IMPROVEMENT

1. Employee Recognition
2. Proper Supervision
3. Recognize Burnout and Job Dissatisfaction
4. Team Building through Decision Making
5. Training
6. Professional Development

When addressing employee recognition, it is important to note that most employees do not feel appreciated for the work they have done. With that said, develop an "Employee if the Month Program." This might seem simple enough, but it is imperative to make it an agenda item at each monthly team meeting where supervisors bring in suggestions and justifications for their nominee. Develop a "Staff Appreciation Board" which is placed in the main room of the program so that staff can thank each other for any assistance they received from other staff members. Employees need to know that they in fact are appreciated.

Supervision is the key element for creating a supportive environment. It is important for the supervisor to always begin staff meetings with positive items and attempt to take out of the conversations, "good/bad" and "right/wrong." These four words are laced in value judgments. Staff value supervisor's education and experience and look to supervisors for knowledge on issues they are dealing with on a daily basis. Supervision should also allow staff a place to vent about their frustrations related to the job.

It is imperative for supervisors to recognize when staff appears to be burning out; when a worker is feeling emotionally exhausted or fatigued, he/she is more likely to withdraw emotionally from their clients. Management plays a key role in making sure that every staff member is taking time off when they feel they are getting burned out.

Utilizing a team approach starts with including all staff in the decision-making process. Staff members want to feel that their opinions and input are important for the treatment of each client; employees who have worked closely with clients need to be involved in the discussion regarding when it is time for a child to be discharged. Asking for feedback from all staff fosters a sense of importance and meaning towards their work. It is also important for supervisors to encourage staff to socialize with each other, as this will assist them in developing a sense of camaraderie and teamwork.

Supervisors need to be sure to provide adequate training that pertains to the population employees are working with and whenever possible provide them with continuing education credit and or certifications. It is important that workers are given time to take classes and that they are given incentives to get further degree as appropriate. In the human services fields, best practices are changing and remaining up-to-date on the latest information and theories can only enhance the workplace in general.

Staff members want to grow professionally, so rewarding loyalty and performance with advancement will add to workers level of satisfaction. If there are no open positions available, create a new title that may reflect the amount of work they are doing and have achieved.

REFERENCES

Agho, A. O., Mueller, C. W., & Price, J. L. (1993). Determinants of employee job satisfaction: An empirical test of a causal model. *Human Relations*, *46*(8): 1007-1027.

Arches, J. (1991). Social structure, burnout, and job satisfaction. *Social Work*, *36*(3): 202-206.

Balfour, D. L. & Neff, D. M. (1993). Predicting and managing turnover in human service agencies: A case study of an organization in crisis. *Public Personnel Management, 22*(3): 473-486.

Blankertz, L. E. & Robinson, S. E. (1997). Turnover intentions of community mental health workers in psychosocial rehabilitation services. *Community Mental Health Journal, 33*(6): 517-531.

Curry, D., McCarragher, T., & Dellmann-Jenkins. M. (2005). Training, transfer, and turnover: Exploring the relationship among transfer of learning factors and staff retention in child welfare. *Children and Youth Services Review,* 27: 931-948.

Decker, J. T., Bailey, T. L., & Westergaard, N. (2002). Burnout among childcare workers, *Residential Treatment for Children and Youth, 19*(4): 61-77

Decker, J. T. (1979). The adolescent alcohol user, misuser and abuser. *The Social Welfare Forum: National Conference on Social Welfare,* 126-138.

Dietzel, L. & Coursey, R. (1998). Predictors of emotional exhaustion among nonresidential staff persons. *Psychiatric Rehabilitation Journal, 21*(4): 340-348.

Ellett, A., & Miller, K. (2004). Professional organizational culture and retention in child welfare: Implications for continuing education for supervision and professional development. *Professional Development: TheInternational Journal of Continuing Social Work Education,* 7: 30-38.

Garland, B. (2002). Prison treatment staff burnout: consequences, causes, and prevention. *Corrections Today,* 116-121.

Hellman, C. M. (1997). Job Satisfaction and Intent to Leave. *The Journal of Social Psychology, 137*(6): 677-689.

Ito, H., Eisen, S. V., Sederer, L. I., Yamada, O., & Tachimori, H. (2001). Factors affecting psychiatric nurses' intention to leave their current job. *Psychiatric Services,* 52(2): 232-234.

Jayaratne, S. (1993). The antecedents, consequences, and correlates of job satisfaction. In R. T. Golembiewski (Ed.) *Handbook of Organizational Behavior* (pp. 111-134). New York: Marcell Dekker.

Kaldenbuerg, D. & Regrut, B. (1999). Do satisfied patients depend on satisfied employees? Or do satisfied employees depend on satisfied patient? *The Satisfaction Monitor,* 3.

Knoop, R. (1995). Work values and job satisfaction. *The Journal of Psychology, 128*(6): 680-693.

Koeske, G. F. & Kirk, S. A. (1995). The effect of characteristics of human service workers on subsequent morale and turnover. *Administration in Social Work, 19*(1): 15-31.

Kreisher, K. (2002). Burn Out. *Child welfare league of America.* Retrieved February 25, 2006 from *www.cwla.org/articles*

Landsman, M. J. (2001). Commitment in public child welfare. *Social Service Review, 75*(3): 386-419

Lum, L., Kervin, J., Clark, K., Reid, F., & Sirola, W. (1998). Explaining nursing turnover intent: Job satisfaction, pay satisfaction, or organizational commitment? *Journal of Organizational Behavior,* 19: 305-320.

Manlove, E. E. & Guzell, J. R. (1997). Intention to leave, anticipated reasons for leaving, and 12-month turnover of child care center staff. *Early Childhood Research Quarterly,* 12: 145-167.

Mor Barak, M. E., Nissly, J. A., & Levin, A. (2001). Antecedents to retention and turn-over among child welfare, social work, and other human service employees: What can we learn from past research? A review and metanalysis. *Social Service Review*, *75*(4): 625-661.

Mor Barak, M. E., Levin, A., Nissly, J. A., & Lane, C. J. (2005). Why do they leave? Modeling child welfare workers' turnover intentions. *Children and Youth Services Review*, *28*(5): 548-577.

Mueller, C. W. & Wallace, J. E. (1996). Justice and the paradox of the contented female worker. *Social Psychology Quarterly*, 59(4): 338-349.

Onyett, S., Phillinger, T., & Muijen, M. (1997). Job satisfaction and burnout among members of community mental health teams. *Journal of Mental Health*, *6*(1): 55-66.

Powell, M. J. & York, R. O. (1992). Turnover in County Public Welfare Agencies. *Journal of Applied Social Sciences*, *16*(2): 111-127.

Regehr, C., Leslie, B., Howe, P., & Chau, S. (2000). Stressors in child welfare practice. *Information for Practice*, 1(2). Web-based journal.

Rose, D., Homes, S., Rose, J., & Hastings, R. (2204). Negative emotional reaction to challenging behavior and staff burnout: two replication studies. *Journal of Applied Research on Intellectual Disabilities*, *17*: 219-223.

Ross, A. (1983). Mitigating turnover of child care staff in group facilities. *Child Welfare*, *62*(1): 63-67.

Seeman, M. (1959). On the meaning of alienation. *American Sociological Review*, *10*(6): 786-787.

Siu, O., Cooper, C. L., & Donald, I. (1997). Occupational stress, job satisfaction and mental health among employees of an acquired TV company in Hong Kong. *Stress Medicine*, 13: 99-107.

Smith, B. (2005). Job retention in child welfare: Effects of perceived organizational support, supervisor support, and intrinsic job value. *Children and Youth Services Review*, 27: 153-169.

Syptak, J., Marsland, D., & Ulmer, D. (1999). Job satisfaction: putting theory into practice. *Retrieved on March 22, 2006 from www, aaafp.org.*

Tett, R. P. & Meyer, J. P. (1993). Job satisfaction, organizational commitment, turnover intention, and turnover: Path analysis based on meta-analytic findings. *Personnel Psychology*, 46: 259-293.

Todd, C. M. & Deery-Schmitt, D. M. (1996). Factors affecting turnover among family child care providers: A longitudinal study. *Early Childhood Research Quarterly*, 11: 351-376.

Tyler, P. & Cushway, D. (1998). Stress and well being in health-care staff: The role of negative affectivity, and perceptions of job demand and discretion. *Stress Medicine*, 14: 99-107.

Weisberg, J. (1994). Measuring worker's burnout and intention to leave. International *Journal of Manpower*, 15(1): 60-71.

Whitaker, K. (1996). Exploring causes of principal burnout. *Journal of Educational Administration*, *34*(1): 60-71.

Whitebook, M., Howes, C., & Phillips, D. (1989). Who cares? Childcare teachers and the quality of care in America. *Oakland CA: Child Care Employee Project.*

APPENDIX A

Questions for the Staff:
What do you like best about your job?

Questions	Not at all	A little	Somewhat	Quite a bit	A lot	Mean
Working with kids						
Team work						
Flexibility						
Freedom						

Open Ended questions related to job satisfaction:

Can you give examples of tasks or responsibilities that make your job meaningful?
What do you like best about your job?
Can you explain how flexibility would be viewed as positive?

What do you like least about job?

Questions	Strongly disagree	A little	Somewhat	Agree	Strongly agree	Mean
Performing restraints on the children						
Hours						
Frequent turnover and lack of staff						
Salary						
Client related issues						

Open Ended questions related to job dissatisfaction, organizational commitment and burnout:

What issues do you feel strongly about that have had a negative effect on your work?
Are there staffing issues that have had a negative effect on your work?
Is financial compensation an issue at this center? Please explain:
Are there issues related to working with clients that we should know about?
What would make your job more satisfying?
What working conditions would improve your level of satisfaction?
When looking at the working environment and whether or not the program encourages teamwork, how would you respond?
Do you feel that management values your work?

APPENDIX B

Questions for the Clients:

Goals Accomplished during Residential Care

Questions	Strongly disagree	A little	Somewhat	Agree	Strongly agree	Mean
Be honest						
Be respectful						
Express yourself appropriately						
Speak up for yourself						
Be a kid						
Focus on yourself						
Listen for the first time						
Learn to follow the house rules						

APPENDIX B (continued)

What are your Feelings and Thoughts on Residential Care

Questions	Not at All	A Little	Some what	Quite a bit	A Lot	Mean
Do you feel that your needs were met at this residence?						
Do you think the staff at this residence respected you?						
Did you respect the program?						
Has the program helped you and your family to get along better?						
Do you think the program staff helped you understand yourself better?						
Do you think you have learned to get along better with others?						
Do you think you will be able to make better choices in the future because of the work you did here?						

Open ended Questions related to goals, accomplishments, feelings and thoughts on residential care

How did you meet the goals of this program?
How do you feel about leaving this program?
Do you have mixed emotions about leaving this program? If yes, what are they?
What could staff do better or differently that would have made your stay here more pleasant?
Did you feel supported by the staff at this facility?
Did the staff give you as much attention as you felt you needed during your stay here?
Did the staff help reunite you with your family?
Did you receive any type of counseling while you were at this facility?

Assessing Staff Competence at Implementing a Multifaceted Residential Program for Youth: Development and Initial Psychometrics of a Staff Observation Form

Kristin Duppong Hurley, PhD
Tanya Shaw, BS
Ron Thompson, PhD
Annette Griffith, MA
Elizabeth M. Farmer, PhD
Jeff Tierney, MEd

INTRODUCTION

Establishing methods for assessing the implementation of services youth receive while in residential care is essential to provide an efficient means for monitoring staff and program performance and determining the effectiveness of residential care interventions. Administrators need to have information to gauge the quality of implementation with regard to staff and programs. Such information may be used to establish the certification of employees or programs and identify the training needs for individual staff or programs. Likewise, the collection of treatment implementation data is crucial to expand the currently limited research base of residential care. Residential care is an essential placement option within the continuum of mental health care for youth; however, the area currently lacks a substantial research foundation regarding its effectiveness (Bates, English, & Kouidou-Giles, 1997; Burns, Hoagwood, & Mrazek, 1999; Curry, 1991; Epstein, 2004; Farmer, Dorsey, & Mustillo, 2004; Frensch & Cameron, 2002; U.S. Department of Health and Human Services, 1999). Among the first steps to prepare for future empirical effectiveness studies is the identification of key treatment ingredients of residential care, constructing operational definitions of these ingredients, and beginning the process of assessing the implementation of these core components in the delivery of services (Curry, 1991; Epstein, 2004; Farmer, 2000; Whittaker, 2004).

Effective implementation of mental health interventions requires the presence of many factors, such as a clearly defined treatment model, staff and administrative support for the intervention, organizational readiness to change, an operationally defined and manualized intervention, effective staff training and supervision, continuous monitoring of program implementation, and a plan for sustainability (Backer, Liberman, & Kuehnel, 1996; Dane & Schneider, 1998; Elliott & Mihalic, 2004; Fixsen, Naoom, Blasé, Friedman, & Wallace, 2005; Torrey et al., 2001). If any of these factors are lacking, the overall implementation of the intervention may be affected. Thus, before one can determine if an intervention is effective, it is crucial to understand how well the program was implemented (Dobson & Cook, 1980; Moncher & Prinz, 1991; Yeaton & Sechrest, 1981). This requires that the intervention have a theory of treatment change, operational definitions of the components of the treatment, and a method for empirically determining the degree to which the intervention was implemented as planned (Chen & Rossi, 1983; Mowbray, Holter, Teague, & Bybee, 2003; Scott & Sechrest, 1989).

While there is increased recognition of the need to monitor the quality of implementation, it is seldom reported in treatment effectiveness studies (Dane & Schneider, 1998; Domitrovich & Greenberg, 2000; Dusenbury, Brannigan, Falco, & Hansen, 2003; Gresham, Gansle, & Noell, 1993; Gottfredson & Gottfredson, 2002; Moncher & Prinz, 1991). Typically, if implementation is discussed in a study, the focus is on the actions the authors took to improve implementation (Dane & Schneider, 1998). It is essential to carry the process one step further and actually assess how well the key treatment ingredients were implemented in order to have any confidence that the treatment strategies were actually put into practice by the service providers.

A rising need within the field of services research is the development of instruments and methods to measure the quality of program implementation to better inform the research-to-practice gap (Bond, Evans, Salyers, Williams, & Kim, 2000; Ginexi & Hilton, 2006). Ideas are just beginning to emerge regarding how to systematically assess treatment fidelity (Bond et al., 2000; Mowbray et al., 2003). Implementation literature in medical (Donabedian, 1966, 1988), behavioral (Fixsen et al., 2005; Scott & Sechrest, 1989), prevention (Dane & Schneider, 1998; Dusenbury, Brannigan, Hansen, Walsh, & Falco, 2005; Mihalic, 2004), and evaluation (Mowbray et al., 2003) fields indicate a variety of frameworks to conceptualize the key concepts related to the quality of program implementation. However, three implementation components are common among the fields: program context, process adherence, and staff competence. First, program context factors, or the measurement of structural variables, refer to the existing administrative organization, caseload ratio, or staff training requirements (Donabedian, 1988; Fixsen et al., 2005). The primary focus of most fidelity work to date has been on the development of measures to assess adherence to structural variables (e.g., training certification, caseloads, and frequency of client contacts) which can be collected fairly reliably and cost-effectively (Mowbray et al., 2003). Second, process adherence is defined as the implementation of core components of the intervention model (Dane & Schneider, 1998; Fixsen et al., 2005). In order to assess this factor, a detailed program theory that operationalizes the core components of the intervention is required. Often, process adherence is measured via observation of staff practices (Dane & Schneider, 1998) but it has also been conducted using surveys of clients and supervisors regarding therapist practices (Henggeler, Schoenwald, Liao, Letourneau, & Edwards, 2002). Process adherence data collection typically is more subjective and expensive to collect, but potentially provides more relevant information on how key aspects of the service were delivered. Third, staff competence goes beyond adherence to consider the quality and skill with which therapists implement the core elements. This includes issues such as staff knowledge, judgment, and enthusiasm for implementing the core components (Donabedian, 1988; Fixsen et al., 2005; Mihalic, 2004). Measures of staff competence require detailed operational definitions of the skill sets required by staff to perform their responsibilities and a system for rating performance. Thus, it is important to recognize the differences between the collection of process and structural information when designing implementation measures.

To date, minimal work has been done to assess the treatment implementation of residential care. We are aware of only two residential care programs that are developing comprehensive program implementation measures. Project Re-Ed has piloted an assessment system for its residential treatment center program (Fields, Farmer, Apperson, Mustillo, & Simmers, 2006; Meadowcroft, Cantrell, & Cantrell, 2002). Girls and Boys Town has also begun a detailed effort to assess information on staff competence implementing an adaptation of the Teaching Family program. This current effort expands upon the existing certification process that has been established for the Teaching Family program (Fixsen, Blasé, Timbers, & Wolf, 2001; Fixsen et al., 2005). Given the urgent questions surrounding the effectiveness of residential care, and that thousands of youth are receiving such care daily, it is of utmost importance to empirically examine the quality of services provided to youth in residential settings and explore the effectiveness of staff support services (training practices, supervision methods, etc.) in these programs as well.

The current study describes the development of an implementation observation system to assess the key process components of a residential program. The focus is on the implementation of key components of an application of the Teaching Family Model such as staff competence implementing token economies, conducting teaching interactions, building relationships with youth, and establishing a youth self-government system (Wolf, Kirigin, Fixsen, Blasé, & Braukmann, 1995). Basic psychometric qualities of the implementation observation form were assessed, including inter-rater agreement and internal consistency of subscales. Predictive validity was assessed by determining if staff members with more years of experience administering the program had higher implementation ratings. An exploratory cluster analysis was also conducted to categorize group-homes in regard to their level of program implementation. This study provides a first step in the development of a comprehensive implementation assessment system to be used by practitioners and researchers interested in understanding the delivery of services to youth in residential care.

METHOD

Program Description

Girls and Boys Town uses an adaptation of the Teaching Family Model called the Family Home Program (Davis & Daly, 2003). Girls and Boys Town is one of the original replication sites of the Teaching Family Model and has been using the approach for over 30 years. The Teaching Family Model is a behaviorally-based residential care approach (Wolf et al., 1976, 1995) with a manualized and well-developed training component (Fixsen et al., 2001) that is currently used in hundreds of adolescent group homes and foster care organizations across the country (Fixsen et al., 2001). The shared goals of the Family Home Program and Teaching Family Model are to improve the behavioral and emotional functioning of youth in a family-style environment by delivering treatment services via married couples living in a home with up to eight youth. The target goals of the intervention are to reduce antisocial behavior, foster the development of social skills, provide youth with positive role models, teach problem-solving techniques, and help youth develop positive relationships with adults and peers. The program utilizes four primary treatment strategies: (1) a token economy; (2) youth self-government system; (3) skill-teaching interactions used by residential couples; and (4) development of mutually rewarding relationships between youth and the residential couples in a family-like setting (Wolf et al., 1995). The Family Home Program emphasizes a systems approach to staff skill development, as well as youth treatment. This involves the integration of training and direct-care staff supervision methods with the evaluation and certification staff. Obtaining reliable model implementation data is critical to this systems integration process.

Participants

Girls and Boys Town employs over 526 residential staff members implementing the Family Home Program in over 11 locations throughout the United States. The study used annual evaluation and certification data collected on residential couples from January 2006 through December 2006. Girls and Boys Town residential staff participate in an annual evaluation system and professional certification process, a requirement for remaining in the position as well as for career advancement. This process includes observations of couples implementing the Family Home Program by program experts and surveys of program administrators. A total of 92 residential couples were observed during 2006. Of these couples, 73% were located on the campus in Boys Town, Nebraska and the remaining 27% were employed at one of 10 different sites throughout the United States. On average, the couples had 3.8 years of experience as a residential couple. However, this is influenced by a handful of couples that were with the program between 10 and 20 years. The median amount of experience was 2.4 years, with 20% of the couples having 12 months or less experience with the residential program.

Measures

Two measures were used in this study, the Staff Implementation Observation Form (SIOF) and program records of staff tenure as residential couples. Each measure is described below.

Staff Implementation Observation Form (SIOF). The SIOF was developed over the course of five years by a variety of program experts from several departments at Girls and Boys Town, including staff training, staff evaluation, research, and residential services. The objective was to create operationally defined items reflecting key aspects of the treatment intervention. The instrument development process began by creating a small team of individuals from the research, staff training, and staff evaluation departments to develop lists of core components of the intervention carried out by residential couples that could easily be observed.

The lists included key components taught in staff training, covered in the treatment manuals, and believed to be essential treatment elements by internal program experts. The topical list included items related to teaching components, self-government, token economies, family-style living, and building youth relationships. The team then reviewed each item, making certain it was not redundant with any other item on the list. Next, item-specific operational definitions of the rating scale anchors were developed. The goal was to go beyond a simple "yes or no" checklist approach and develop a five-point rating scale to assess finer shades of implementation. The five-point scale included the implementation choices of "no/incorrect, below average, average, above average, and excellent." Detailed operational definitions were developed for the "no/incorrect, average, and excellent" rating anchors. After the items and corresponding definitions were developed, they were reviewed by internal program experts to determine if any key elements needed to be added and to improve the wording of existing items. After revisions, the items were then reviewed by program administrators and supervisors for clarity and again revised. The instrument was then pilot tested to determine the feasibility of assessing each concept during in-home observations. This iterative process of testing, revising, and redistributing the instrument occurred repeatedly over the course of three years, resulting in the development of an observational instrument with 63 items. A Users Guide to accompany the instrument was also created, which includes specific anchor definitions (no/incorrect, average, and excellent) for each item.

From the 63-item observation form, 26 high-frequency items (easy to rate during a 60-90 minute observation) were selected to be piloted by the evaluation and certification department beginning in January 2006. The 26 items in the SIOF reflect the key elements of the model: staff competence implementing token economies (6 items), conducting teaching interactions (7 items), building relationships and family-style environments with youth (7 items), and establishing a youth self-government system (6 items). Two samples of items and definitions for the anchors are provided in Figure 1.

Staff experience. Staff experience was measured by obtaining the number of months from the date of hire as a residential couple to the date the SIOF was conducted. As considerable variance in the range of staff experience was expected, we created a categorical variable of staff experience with four levels, less than 12 months (under a year experience), 12-23 months (in the second year), 24 to 50 months (a few years of experience), and 51 or more months (long-term residential couples).

FIGURE 1. Two Sample Items from the Staff Implementation Observation Form, Including the Item-Stem and Definitions for the No/Incorrect, Average, and Excellent Rating Anchors

---

A. Gives preventive prompts and/or social cues to youth

   (1) No/Incorrect: Absence of prompts/cues, or use of prompts/cues when proactive teaching was necessary.

   (2) Below Average:

   (3) Average: Recognizes and acts on most opportunities to use preventive prompts. Prompts typically surround events.

   (4) Above Average:

   (5) Excellent: Prompting is part of natural conversation with youth (e.g. not only surrounding teaching). Prompting is reinforcing to youth and supportive in tone. Spontaneously gives prompts as part of the natural routine.

B. Encourages youth to engage in positive interactions with peers

   (1) No/Incorrect: Misses opportunities to teach positive peer relationships. Does not handle peer conflict well or does not teach to it competently.

   (2) Below Average:

   (3) Average: Encourages youth to engage in positive interactions with peers, such as how to get along with others and how to respect each other. Models positive peer interactions.

   (4) Above Average:

   (5) Excellent: Spontaneously teaches youth how to be good siblings and friends with each other. actively teaches positive peer modeling and peer coaching.

Procedures

The process for completing the implementation observation form included pairs of trained observers going into the residential home for 60-120 minutes to observe natural interactions among the residential couples and youth. All of the observers were employees of Girls and Boys Town, were highly skilled in implementation of the residential program, and were either program supervisors or members of the staff evaluation department. Prior to beginning the observation, the observer was trained on the observation form and the Users Guide with specific definitions for each item. A detailed 3-hour training, which included a review of the purpose of the assessment instrument, instructions on how to rate each item, and practice scoring items based on the review of videos was conducted with 73% of the observers. The remaining 27% of observers received an abbreviated training conducted by staff evaluation personnel. Each observation was conducted by two individuals who observed residential homes during periods of high interaction between staff and youth (i.e., after school). Each home was observed once. Following the observation, evaluators independently rated the implementation of key model elements using an electronic version of the 26-item SIOF, which allowed for the immediate tallying of subscale scores and preparation of graphs indicating the relative strengths and weaknesses of each residential couple.

All of the archival data for this study were compiled by researchers at Girls and Boys Town and all information that could identify residential couples were removed from the dataset. Basic psychometric analyses of the SIOF were conducted, including inter-rater agreement and internal consistency of subscales. Predictive validity of the SIOF was assessed by determining if staff members with more years of experience administering the program had higher implementation ratings. An exploratory cluster analysis was also conducted to categorize group-homes in regard to their level of program implementation.

RESULTS

Inter-Rater Agreement Analyses and Internal Consistency

Initial analyses involving 92 observations in group homes conducted by pairs of observers indicated acceptable inter-rater agreement. The observations were conducted by 36 different observers. Four primary observers from the staff evaluation department were involved in rating 91% of the observations, 52% of the time a member of staff evaluation was accompanied by a program supervisor, and 39% of the time two staff evaluation members conducted the observation. In 9% of the observations two program supervisors conducted the evaluation, with no one from the staff evaluation department participating in the observation. Inter-rater agreement was examined for perfect agreement and agreement within one rating point. For perfect agreement, an agreement rating of 70% or higher is desired (Stemler, 2004). For the entire 26-item scale, the observers had perfect agreement 76% of the time, with 99.5% agreement within one rating point. The subscales ranged from 74.1 to 81.1% perfect agreement and 99.3 to 100% to agreement within one point. The lowest level of perfect agreement was 65.2% for one item. All other items had 70% perfect inter-rater agreement or higher. An intraclass correlation coefficient was calculated using the one-way random effects model comparing the overall mean implementation score given by each rater. Overall, the intraclass correlation coefficient was .93, $F(91, 92) = 26.49$, $p < .001$, indicating a strong correlation between the ratings of the pair of observers. Despite the small number of items in each subscale, the internal consistency Cronbach's Alpha coefficients were high, ranging from a low of .83 for the Self-Government subscale to a high of .95 for the Relationships subscale.

Item-Level Scale Descriptives

As shown in Table 1, the 26 items in the SIOF have mean scores near 3.0 and reasonable distributions. Across all 26 items, the mean score was 3.20 with a standard deviation of .70. The distribution of scores (based on the averaged scores between two observers) indicated that about 17% of scores on an individual item had "low implementation" (scores between 1.0 and 2.4), 42% "average implementation" (scores between 2.5 and 3.4) and 37% "high implementation" (scores between 3.5 and 5.0). Overall, the two highest-scoring items involved relationship-building items "maintains quality components" (mean = 3.57) and "expressing interest in the happiness and well-being of each youth" (mean = 3.53). The two lowest scoring items were "encourages use of problem solving strategies where warranted" (mean = 2.80) and "uses corrective teaching in response to inappropriate behaviors" (mean = 2.82). Looking at the subscales, one can see that the Relationship subscale had the highest overall score (mean score of 3.38 and 44.6% of observations with high implementation scores) and the Self-Government subscale had the lowest overall score (mean score of 3.02 and 15.2% of observations with high implementation scores).

Predictive Validity

A one-way multivariate analysis of variance (MANOVA) was conducted to determine the relationship between four levels of staff experience (less than 12 months, 12 to 23 months, 24 to 50 months, and greater than 51 months) and staff implementation ratings on each scale of the SIOF. Significant differences were found across the four categories of experience on the SIOF scale ratings, Wilk's Lambda = 0.66, $F(3, 88) = 3.19$, $p < .001$. As the overall MANOVA was significant, analyses of variance (ANOVA) on each rating scale were conducted as follow-up tests. Each of the ANOVA analyses were significant, indicating that there were significant differences across the different staff experience

TABLE 1. Staff Implementation Observation (SIOF) Item Means, Standard Deviations, Sample Sizes, and Score Distributions

SIOF Item	M (sd)	n	% Scores 1.0-2.4 (Low)	% Scores 2.5-3.4 (Average)	% Scores 3.5-5.0 (High)
Teaching Components Items					
Sets appropriate tolerances for behaviors	3.08 (.65)	92	25.0	41.3	33.7
Provides specific descriptions of youth behavior	3.09 (.71)	92	21.7	46.7	31.5
Teaches correct/ appropriate skills based on youth behaviors	3.23 (.69)	92	15.2	43.5	41.3
Gives preventive prompts and/or social cues to youth	3.26 (.81)	92	21.7	29.3	48.9
Uses effective praise to reinforce appropriate youth behaviors	3.21 (.79)	92	21.7	38.0	40.2
Uses corrective teaching in response to inappropriate behaviors	2.82 (.70)	92	35.6	45.6	18.9
Uses rationales to generalize social skills to other situations	3.14 (.75)	92	27.2	32.6	40.2
Teaching Components Subscale	3.12 (.61)	92	18.5	53.3	28.3
Token Economy Items					
Teaches to individual target skills	3.17 (.74)	92	19.6	39.1	41.3
Teaching interactions include consequences	3.32 (.58)	92	7.6	50.0	42.4
Delivers positive and negative consequences fairly	3.12 (.64)	92	20.7	45.7	33.7
Makes privileges contingent on youth behavior	3.28 (.60)	92	10.9	43.5	45.7
Appropriately utilizes Motivation System special conditions	3.18 (.55)	91	9.9	58.2	31.9
Motivates youth to advance Motivation Systems	3.25 (.65)	91	8.8	52.7	38.5
Token Economy Subscale	3.22 (.51)	92	7.6	62.0	30.4

Continued

TABLE 1. (continued)

SIOF Item	M (sd)	n	% Scores 1.0-2.4 (Low)	% Scores 2.5-3.4 (Average)	% Scores 3.5-5.0 (High)
Relationship Building Items					
Expresses interest in the happiness and well-being of each youth	3.53 (.80)	92	13.0	25.0	62.0
Maintains quality components	3.57 (.80)	92	10.9	30.4	58.7
Staff model and/or teach relationship-building skills to youth	3.38 (.80)	92	14.1	39.1	46.7
Converses naturally with youth at meals, during activities, etc.	3.37 (.85)	92	14.1	35.9	50.0
Readily shares youth accomplishments with visitors to the home	3.29 (.83)	92	18.5	37.0	44.6
Balances youth relationship building with teaching	3.19 (.73)	92	20.7	41.3	38.0
Encourages youth to engage in positive interactions with peers	3.33 (.73)	92	10.9	42.4	46.7
Relationship Building Subscale	3.38 (.70)	92	10.9	44.6	44.6
Self Government Items					
Encourages use of problem solving strategies where warranted	2.80 (.68)	92	33.7	48.9	17.4
Reinforces/encourages use of reporting systems	3.13 (.51)	90	10.0	61.1	28.9
Follows an established process in self-government meetings	3.11 (.65)	92	19.6	46.7	33.7
Self-government meetings provide quality opportunities for youth input and decision making	3.00 (.67)	92	25.0	45.7	29.3
Implements youth leadership system	3.11 (.59)	92	14.1	54.3	31.5
Implements Appeals Process	2.97 (.60)	91	23.1	56.0	20.9
Self Government Subscale	3.02 (.46)	92	17.4	67.4	15.2

groups on each of the SIOF subscales (see Table 2). A post hoc analysis for each univariate ANOVA was done using the Scheffe method, to examine the differences in significance for each level of experience. Across all four subscales, the post hoc analyses indicated that staff in the higher experience group obtained higher SIOF rating scores than those in the lower experience group.

Ability to Discriminate Implementation Scores for Individual Residential Homes

An exploratory cluster analysis of the 26 items on the SIOF was used to differentiate implementation patterns among the individual group homes. The analysis to cluster group homes based on their SIOF implementation scores was conducted using the Ward's linkage method and the squared Euclidean distance measure with solutions ranging from 8 to 2 clusters. A large jump in the dissimilarity coefficients occurred between the three and two cluster solutions, suggesting that a three cluster solution may best categorize the group homes. As shown in Table 3, the mean implementation scores for each subscale were the lowest for cluster one, average for cluster two, and the highest for cluster three. The largest numbers of group homes were in the lowest performing cluster, followed by the average performing cluster with the fewest

TABLE 2. ANOVA Results for Staff Length of Experience by Implementation Subscale

	Less than 12 months n = 17	12 to 23 months n = 22	24 to 50 months n = 28	More than 51 months n = 25	Total	ANOVA
	M (sd)	M (sd)	M (sd)	M (sd)	M (sd)	F
Teaching[a,b]	2.71 (.39)	2.99 (.59)	3.14 (.60)	3.50 (.54)	3.12 (.61)	7.59*
Token Economy[a,b]	2.90 (.39)	3.02 (.48)	3.26 (.46)	3.55 (.48)	3.21 (.51)	8.41*
Self Government[a,b,c]	2.65 (.37)	2.88 (.35)	3.08 (.38)	3.32 (.46)	3.02 (.46)	11.05*
Relationships[a,b,c]	2.91 (.54)	3.12 (.64)	3.45 (.69)	3.84 (.56)	3.38 (.70)	9.23*

Note. Significant differences at $p < .05$ using post-hoc Scheffe pairwise comparisons are indicated with subscripts.
[a] = significant difference from "less than 12 months" and "greater than 51 months."
[b] = significant difference from "less than 12 months" and "24 to 50 months."
[c] = significant difference from "12 to 23 months" and "greater than 51 months."
* $p < .001$.

TABLE 3. Three Exploratory Clusters and Their Implementation Scores for Each SIOF Subscale

	Cluster 1 (Low) n = 41	Cluster 2 (Average) n = 30	Cluster 3 (High) n = 21
SIOF Subscale	M (sd)	M (sd)	M (sd)
Relationship Building	2.79 (0.49)	3.57 (0.25)	4.25 (0.29)
Self-Government	2.63 (0.29)	3.15 (0.19)	3.58 (0.27)
Teaching Components	2.62 (0.38)	3.26 (0.19)	3.91 (0.40)
Token Economy	2.80 (0.31)	3.35 (0.31)	3.84 (0.26)

group homes in the highest implementing cluster. This three cluster solution of low, average, and high implementing group homes was selected as the most useful categorization of homes by implementation scores.

This three cluster solution was examined in relationship to the extent of staff experience for the residential couples. An ANOVA between cluster membership and staff experience was significant $F(2, 89) = 25.77$, $p < .001$, indicating that staff tenure did differ by low, average, or high cluster membership. Staff experience increased as implementation quality of the cluster improved. Post hoc Scheffe tests indicated that there was a significant difference between the low-implementation group and the high-implementation group ($p < .001$), and between the low-implementation group and the average-implementation group ($p < .001$).

DISCUSSION

The purpose of this study was to determine if observers would be able to reliably differentiate implementation performance among trained couples serving youth in residential care. The initial results for the 26-item Staff Implementation Observation Form (SIOF) suggest that it may be a promising approach for assessing treatment implementation by staff in residential settings. This study examined inter-rater agreement and internal scale consistency, predictive validity, scale-descriptives and distributions, and the ability to differentiate similar groups of staff implementation. First, the inter-rater agreement rates and internal scale consistency scores were acceptable. It appears that trained observers can reliably conduct the observation, with 76% perfect agreement across all items and all observers. This is especially encouraging, as the study utilized

36 observers, and still was able to maintain high inter-rater agreement rates. The high internal consistency scores suggest that the subscale items are assessing similar constructs.

Second, there is evidence of predictive validity, as the SIOF was related to the years of experience for the residential couples. This finding, that as implementation scores increased so did staff tenure, suggests that the SIOF is capable of predicting constructs related to staff implementation. However, future studies would benefit from tracking the implementation scores of staff over time to determine if the SIOF could be utilized to predict the likelihood of staff retention. Moreover, tracking staff implementation scores over time would allow for the prediction of patterns of implementation change and perhaps the identification of high, average, and low growth in treatment implementation skills.

Third, looking at the SIOF items, the mean score for each item was at or slightly above or below 3.0 on a five-point scale, or otherwise "average." The two highest scoring items involved relationship-building items, suggesting that residential couples were most skilled at relating to youth. The two lowest scoring items were "encourages use of problem-solving strategies where warranted" (mean = 2.80) and "uses corrective teaching in response to inappropriate behaviors" (mean = 2.82). This suggests that some of the technical components of teaching skills to youth require additional skill development. Also, these are among the skills that administrators report taking the most time to develop. So, the low implementation scores in these areas may reflect the ongoing skill acquisition of less-experienced residential couples.

In addition to looking at the mean-item scores, it is important to look at the item distributions. The SIOF instrument was designed to encourage the use of the entire 5-point range, as appropriate. The distributions indicated a majority of scores occurred in the middle of the scale, with a substantial 20-30% of scores in the high range and 15-20% in the low range. The item-level distributions suggest that observers were using the entire 5-point range of the scale. When implementing a multifaceted intervention it may take months, if not years, for staff to implement the program masterfully. So, having a range of implementation scores is expected. Thus, the SIOF assessment approach clearly helps to identify the exceptional instances of implementation and those that need additional training assistance. Having a five-point rating scale provided an ability to discriminate between levels of implementation competence, and should help program administrators identify staff training needs and monitor staff performance over time. Moreover, we suspect that the presence of detailed definitions, explaining the low, middle, and high anchors for each definition and the training process that accompanies the observation form were instrumental in assisting in the reliability of the inter-rater observations. With the presence of descriptions of the observed behavior for each item, we are more confident that the ratings reflect actual staff implementation.

Fourth, the study was designed to examine if this observational implementation approach would be able to discriminate implementation levels among residential group homes. While it might be able to detect differences on individual items in the scale, it is also useful to practitioners if it can also identify staff with overall low and high implementation. The analyses in Table 1 focus on the distribution of scores by individual items. This analysis focuses on integrating the information from all 26 items into a classification of group homes. Using an exploratory cluster analysis of homes with the 26 items of the SIOF, we found the presence of three distinct groups of implementers, low, average, and high. As shown in Table 3, the largest group was comprised of the low implementers. Even for the lowest performing group, the average implementation scores were between 2.62 and 2.80 on the subscales. The high implementation group had mean subscale scores of 3.58 to 4.25, which is quite impressive. This finding of distinct groups of implementers suggests that there are groups of residential couples that tend to score consistently lower, about average, or higher across the 26-item scale. It is important to keep in mind that there was variation within each subgroup of implementation (see minimum and maximum scores on Table 3). While the mean subscale score is low for the low implementation group, there were individuals in the low implementation group that would have higher implementation scores on individual items. The clustering technique maximizes differences among the clusters, so one can think of the couples in the low implementation group as scoring lower overall than the couples in the other two classification groups. This approach of classifying group homes is useful for identifying which staff members may need additional training or supervision support.

Of special interest for supervisors is to examine the subscale and individual-item scores for couples to determine the respective areas of strength and areas for individual improvement. These three groups had varying rates of experience as residential couples, with the low implementation group having the least amount of experience and the highest implementers having the most years of experience with the intervention. This finding that implementation rates improve with increased experience fits with the rather high learning curve that accompanies a comprehensive treatment model for living with youth in an intensive, family-style environment. It also is probable that staff with continuous low implementation scores will be more likely to leave the organization earlier (either voluntary or involuntary) than those implementing the program successfully. It will be interesting for future studies to examine the change trajectories for implementation rates over time, to examine if there is a difference between implementation growth rates for staff that stay with the program or leave after one or two years.

Limitations

The small sample size of this pilot study limited the ability to run additional analyses, such as confirmatory factor analyses. Future studies will need to be conducted to replicate the findings of this pilot study and confirm the factor structure of the SIOF. In addition to the limitation of the small sample size, the study was not able to assess the test-retest reliability by conducting multiple observations of a residential couple in a close proximity of time. Further, this study was not able to conduct multiple implementation assessments over time to assess the ability of the instrument to measure changes in implementation. This lack of multiple assessments limited the predictive utility of the instrument. Hopefully future studies will be able to examine the ability of the instrument to assess change in implementation rates over time. Finally, this study did not have access to multiple measures of implementation quality to examine convergent validity. Future studies would benefit from the inclusion of assessments from other sources that examine similar implementation constructs to examine convergent and predictive validity.

Recommendations

This approach of examining different implementation patterns among staff is a key direction for future research studies on service delivery issues in residential care. In the exploratory cluster analyses, initially some very extreme clusters formed and gradually merged into the final three clusters of low, middle, and high implementation. With larger sample sizes, one may be able to look at cluster analyses with more differentiated groups than just the three broad clusters of low, middle, and high implementation, and thus identify more unique implementation styles. For example, it will be interesting to investigate if there are different patterns of implementation, such as staff with high relationship implementation but low teaching implementation or low relationships but high self-government implementation. By assessing a variety of components of the treatment model, researchers will be able to examine if particular patters of implementation begin to emerge for staff. Likewise, it may be that certain staff follow different trajectories of implementation, starting lower or higher in certain constructs and then growing over time.

Moreover, it will be interesting to see if staff implementation rates are related to youth outcomes. A frequent finding in the literature is that higher implementation will relate to improved youth outcomes (Dane & Schneider, 1998; Domitrovich & Greenberg, 2000; Mihalic, 2004). However, we are aware of only one study of residential programs for youth, conducted on the Teaching Family Model, which found a relationship between increased talking and proximity between family teachers and youth and a decrease in youth-reported delinquency (Solnick, Braukmann, Bedlington, Kirigin, & Wolf, 1981). Hopefully this implementation assessment approach will begin to assist future studies to examine the role of implementation on youth outcomes. It may even be able to identify if certain patterns of implementation are most critical to obtain positive youth outcomes.

Future research would also benefit from including multiple assessments of implementation, including program context, process adherence, and staff competence. The three approaches collect information on different facets of program implementation and are useful for understanding treatment integrity (Dane & Schneider, 1998; Mihalic, 2004). However, research needs to be conducted to examine the differences among these types of treatment fidelity data sources and determine how they can each be best utilized to improve program implementation and systems functioning. For example, it may be that fidelity assessments focused on program adherence and staff competence would be the most useful for supervisors of residential programs as they provide detailed implementation information that can vary considerably by individual staff members. It may also be that some forms of treatment fidelity assessments are more predictive of youth outcomes. For example, there may be little variance on program context factors (i.e., staff-to-youth ratios), so the more variable staff competence components may be better predictors of client outcomes. By including comprehensive and multifaceted treatment fidelity measures, future research will be able to learn much more about the quality of treatment implementation in residential care as well as refining training and supervision models.

Finally, although it took a considerable amount of time to develop the initial observation items and definitions and pilot initial versions, this process was instrumental in developing an assessment approach that can be reliably used by staff. The act of involving a variety of different organizational departments to be part of the instrument development process increased overall agency buy-in and support for the effort to assess implementation. Further, creating an instrument that had a variety of applications, such as immediate feedback for supervisors to use with individual direct-care staff and the ability to aggregate the data and examine program trends over time, added to the utility of using such an assessment approach. The multiple iterations of the instrument, participation from a variety of inter-agency departments, and involvement of a wide range of staff from direct-care providers to upper-level administrators helped to create a comprehensive implementation measure that could be readily used in an applied setting.

CONCLUSIONS

This pilot study of an observation-based implementation assessment scale of staff competence delivering a multifaceted intervention shows initial promise. The scale demonstrated reasonable psychometric properties. Moreover, the instrument allows administrators the ability to examine the item-level implementation of individual staff members in order to identify the specific training needs within each subscale, allowing a more fine-tuned approach to staff development efforts. Thus, from a practitioner perspective, the SIOF appears to offer a promising approach for assessing staff implementation of a complex treatment model in residential care. Future research is needed to replicate these results, determine the relationship between more intricate implementation patterns of the intervention, examine changes in staff implementation competence over time, and investigate the relationship between staff implementation and youth outcomes.

REFERENCES

Backer, T. E., Liberman, R. P., & Kuehnel, T. G. (1996). Dissemination and adoption of innovative psychosocial interventions. *Journal of Consulting and Clinical Psychology, 54*(1), 111-118.

Bates, B., English, D., & Kouidou-Giles, S. (1997). Residential treatment and its alternatives: A review of the literature. *Child and Youth Care Forum, 26*, 7-51.

Bond, G. R., Evans, L., Salyers, M. P., Williams, J., & Kim, H. (2000). Measurement of fidelity in psychiatric rehabilitation. *Mental Health Services Research, 2*, 75-87.

Burns, B. J., Hoagwood, K., & Mrazek, P. J. (1999). Effective treatment for mental disorders in children and adolescents. *Clinical Child and Family Psychology Review, 2*, 199-254.

Chen, H., & Rossi, P. H. (1983). Evaluating with sense: The theory-driven approach. *Evaluation Review, 7,* 283-302.

Curry, J. F. (1991). Outcome research on residential treatment: Implications and suggested directions. *American Journal of Orthopsychiatry, 61,* 348-357.

Dane, A. V., & Schneider, B. H. (1998). Program integrity in primary and early secondary prevention: Are implementation effects out of control? *Clinical Psychology Review, 18,* 23-45.

Davis, J., & Daly, D. L. (2003). *Long-Term Residential Program Training Manual, 4th Edition.* Boys Town, Nebraska: Father Flanagan's Boy's Home.

Dobson, D., & Cook, T. J. (1980). Avoiding type III error in program evaluation: Results from a field experiment. *Evaluation and Program Planning, 3,* 269-276.

Domitrovich, C. E., & Greenberg, M. T. (2000). The study of implementation: Current findings from effective programs that prevent mental disorders in school-aged children. *Journal of Educational and Psychological Consultation, 71,* 193-221.

Donabedian, A. (1966). Evaluating the quality of medical care. *The Milbank Memorial Fund Quarterly, 44,* 166-203.

Donabedian, A. (1988). The quality of care: How can it be assessed? *Journal of the American Medical Association, 260,* 1743-1748.

Dusenbury, L., Brannigan, R., Falco, M., & Hansen, W. B. (2003). A review of research on fidelity of implementation: Implications for drug abuse prevention in school settings. *Health Education Research, 18,* 237-256.

Dusenbury, L., Brannigan, R., Hansen, W. B., Walsh, J., & Falco, M. (2005). Quality of implementation: Developing measures crucial to understanding the diffusion of preventive interventions. *Health Education Research, 20,* 308-313.

Elliott, D. S., & Mihalic, S. (2004). Issues in disseminating and replicating effective prevention programs. *Prevention Science, 5,* 47-53.

Epstein, R. A., Jr. (2004). Inpatient and residential treatment effects for children and adolescents: A review and critique. *Child and Adolescent Psychiatric Clinics of North America, 13,* 411-428.

Farmer, E. M. Z. (2000). Issues confronting effective services in systems of care. *Children and Youth Services Review, 22*(8), 627-650.

Farmer, E. M. Z., Dorsey, S., & Mustillo, S. A. (2004). Intensive home and community interventions. *Child and Adolescent Psychiatric Clinics of North America, 13*(4), 857-884.

Fields, E., Farmer, E. M. Z., Apperson, J., Mustillo, S., & Simmers, D. (2006). Treatment and posttreatment effects of residential treatment using a re-education model. *Behavioral Disorders, 31,* 312-322.

Fixsen, D. L., Blase, K. A., Timbers, G. D., & Wolf, M. M. (2001). In search of program implementation: 729 replications of the teaching-family model. In G. A. Bernfeld, D. P. Farrington, & A. W. Leschied (Eds.), *Offender Rehabilitation in Practice* (pp. 149-166). New York: John Wiley & Sons, Ltd.

Fixsen, D. L., Naoom, S. F., Blasé, K. A., Friedman, R. M., & Wallace, F. (2005). *Implementation research: A synthesis of the literature. Tampa,* FL: University of South Florida, Louis de la Parte Florida Mental Health Institute, The National Implementation Research Network (FMHI Publication #231).

Frensch, K. M., & Cameron, G. (2002). Treatment of choice or a last resort? A review of residential mental health placements for children and youth. *Child and Youth Care Forum, 31*, 307-339.

Ginexi, E. M., & Hilton, T. F. (2006). What's next for translational research? *Evaluation & the Health Profession, 29*, 334-347.

Gottfredson, D. C., & Gottfredson, G. D. (2002). Quality of school-based prevention programs: Results from a national survey. *Journal of Research in Crime and Delinquency, 39*, 3-35.

Gresham, F. M., Gansle, K. A., & Noell, G. H. (1993). Treatment integrity in applied behavior analysis with children. *Journal of Applied Behavior Analysis, 26*, 257-263.

Henggeler, S. W., Schoenwald, S. K., Liao, J. G., Letourneau, E. J., & Edwards, D. L. (2002). Transporting efficacious treatments to field settings: The link between supervisory practices and therapist fidelity in MST programs. *Journal of Clinical Psychology, 31*, 155-167.

Meadowcroft, P., Cantrell, M. L., & Cantrell, R. P. (2002). Measuring the fidelity of Re-ED programs. *Reclaiming Children and Youth: Journal of Strength-based Interventions, 11*(2), 116-119.

Mihalic, S. (2004). The importance of implementation fidelity. *Emotional & Behavioral Disorders in Youth, 4*, 83-86, 99-105.

Moncher, F., & Prinz, R. (1991). Treatment fidelity in outcome studies. *Clinical Psychology Review, 11*, 247-266.

Mowbray, C. T., Holter, M. C., Teague, G. B., & Bybee, D. (2003). Fidelity criteria: Development, measurement, and validation. *American Journal of Education, 24*, 315-340.

Scott, A. G., & Sechrest, L. (1989). Strength of theory and theory of strength. *Evaluation and Program Planning, 12*, 329-336.

Solnick, J. V., Braukmann, C. J., Bedlington, M. M., Kirigin, K. A., & Wolf, M. M. (1981). The relationship between parent-youth interaction and delinquency in group homes. *Journal of Abnormal Child Psychology, 9*, 107-119.

Stemler, S. E. (2004). A comparison of consensus, consistency, and measurement approaches to estimating interrater reliability. *Practical Assessment, Research & Evaluation, 9(4)*. Retrieved April 4, 2007 from http://PAREonline.net/getvn.asp?v=9&n=4.

Torrey, W. C., Drake, R. E., Dixon, L., Burns, B. J., Flynn, L., Rush, A. J., et al. (2001). Implementing evidence-based practices for persons with severe mental illnesses. *Psychiatric Services, 54*, 45-50.

U.S. Department of Health and Human Services. (1999). *Mental Health: A Report of the Surgeon General.* Rockville, MD: U.S. Department of Health and Human Services, Substance Abuse and Mental Health Services Administration, Center for Mental Health Services, National Institutes of Health, National Institute of Mental Health.

Whittaker, J. K. (2004). The re-invention of residential treatment: An agenda for research and practice. *Child and Adolescent Psychiatry Clinics of North America, 13*, 267-278.

Wolf, M. M., Kirigin, K. A., Fixsen, D. L., Blasé, K. A., & Braukmann, C. J. (1995). The teaching-family model: A case study in data-based program development and refinement (and dragon wrestling). *Journal of Organizational Behavior Management, 15,* 11-68.

Wolf, M. M., Phillips, E., Fixsen, D., Baukmann, C. J., Kirigin, K. A., Willner, A. G., et al. (1976). Achievement Place: The Teaching-Family Model. *Child Care Quarterly, 5,* 92-103.

Yeaton, W. H., & Sechrest, L. (1981). Critical dimensions in choice and maintenance of successful treatments: Strength, integrity, and effectiveness. *Journal of Consulting and Clinical Psychology, 49*(2), 156-167.

Assessment of Behavior Management and Behavioral Interventions in State Child Welfare Facilities

Stephen E. Wong, PhD

INTRODUCTION

Recent research indicates that nearly half of the children entering this nation's child welfare system have serious emotional and behavioral disorders (Burns et al., 2004). These behavioral disorders can be manifested in dangerous acts such as physical aggression, self-injury, property destruction, or highly disruptive behavior. Behaviors of this sort present at least two challenges to residential treatment facilities that care for these youth. The first challenge is finding acceptable methods of behavior management to keep the children from harming themselves or others, as well as minimizing damage and disorder to the living unit. The second challenge is in finding effective treatments or ways of modifying children's conduct and reducing future occurrences of problem behavior.

Behavioral interventions, procedures for increasing prosocial behavior and decreasing undesired behavior derived from principles of operant and social learning theory, offer evidence-based treatments to meet the second challenge (Wong, in press). Behavioral interventions include providing children with rationales and specific guidelines for desired behavior, teaching social and functional skills, setting attainable criteria for clients' performance and gradually raising these criteria, providing positive reinforcement (e.g., praise, tokens exchangeable for extra privileges, activities, or snacks) to motivate desired behavior, and administering mild reductive consequences (e.g., temporary loss of extra privileges) to discourage inappropriate behavior. Properly designed behavioral programs also incorporate data collection systems to monitor clients' performance to ensure that presumed positive reinforcement is operating as such, and that progress is being made toward intended goals.

A number of authors have written about the feasibility of behavioral programs for residential treatment facilities and reported favorable outcomes associated with their use. Nabors et al. (2003) described the successful application of behavioral management procedures in a summer program for homeless children. Lietz (2004) discussed advantages of combining reinforcement contingencies with a social learning milieu to address severe behavior problems in children and adolescents in a residential treatment facility. In a review paper, Foltz (2004) noted that behavioral interventions can be as efficacious as psychotropic medications in dealing with behavior problems in youth with Attention Deficit-Hyperactivity Disorder (ADHD) and produce more durable gains. Behavioral interventions have also been associated with reductions in violent incidents against others and self, runaways, and other misbehavior in youth in short-term emergency shelters (Hurley, Ingram, Czyz, Juliano, & Wilson, 2006), and with reductions in severe aggression, self-injury, property destruction, and other serious inappropriate behavior in adolescents undergoing long-term psychiatric hospitalization and residential treatment (Wong, 1999). In a controlled study with delinquent youth randomly assigned to either intensive foster care with behavioral programming or to a typical group home placement, intensive foster care was shown to be more effective in reducing the frequency of arrests, incarcerations, and runways (Chamberlain & Moore, 1998).

Although behavioral interventions would appear to be a beneficial component of residential treatment, there is little data on the extent to which they are being utilized or the exact manner in which they are being applied in these facilities. Murray and Sefchik (1992) suggested that carefully written state regulations based on published research should guide the correct usage of behavioral procedures. This, in turn, could lead to the implementation of more humane and effective residential programs. However, these authors did not assess either agencies' adherence to promulgated regulations or the actual quality of behavioral treatment for children and youth in residential care.

The present study examined the usage of behavioral interventions in one state's child welfare substitute-care facilities. Program reviews of all state-funded agencies over a 10-year period were analyzed to assess the types of behavioral procedures being used and the degree to which current agency practices conformed to established principles of learning theory. Data were also collected on the type and number of professional staff available on site to implement and oversee these procedures.

METHOD

Compliance Reviews

This study was based on the analysis of official reports generated by the Office of Program Review (OPR). The OPR was a unit within the Department of Children and Families of a highly populated Midwestern state. Programs reviewed by the OPR included foster care agencies, group homes, and institutions, but not home-of-relative foster care placements. This study examined OPR "compliance reviews" or the most intensive reviews routinely conducted by this office. These evaluations were scheduled every 3-5 years and emulated program reviews of the Joint Commission for Accreditation of Healthcare Organizations. Reviews included interviews with state personnel who interacted with the agency; on-site inspection and interviews with facility administrators, clinicians, direct care staff, and clients; and examination of institutional policy and procedures, clinical program descriptions, operation logs, and individual client records. OPR reviewers had bachelors or master's degrees in social sciences and work experience in social service agencies, and their review of an agency culminated with a written report. A state official who had assumed the responsibilities for the OPR gave the present author access to all OPR compliance reviews performed during the years of 1984-94. During this 10-year period all 204 private agencies contracting with the state to provide substitute care underwent at least one review.

One portion of the review process examined agency discipline and behavior management procedures to see if they were in compliance with state regulations and licensing requirements. Like many other states, this state prohibited the use of corporal punishment, verbal abuse, and mechanical restraint, as well as procedures that would infringe on clients' basic needs and rights, such as access to meals, sleep, clothing, and visits with family. State regulations also limited the duration of privilege removal, restriction to one's room or the facility, and physical confinement or seclusion as forms of behavior management. Inspection of discipline and behavior management procedures was embedded within an overall review of agencies' clinical program, staff ratios and qualifications, organizational policy and structure, physical plant, and daily operation.

Scoring and Analysis of Compliance Reviews

Two research assistants, both social work graduate students, read the official compliance reviews to quantify various features of the substitute care programs. Research assistants referred to written definitions of behavioral procedures to score the presence or absence of these procedures in the agency program descriptions. They also used the comprehensive compliance reviews to count the type and number of professional staff working at each facility.

Behavioral Procedures. To analyze and quantify agency behavioral interventions, each compliance review was scored for the presence of 14 behavioral procedures within three categories: (1) restrictive procedures or reductive consequences that might be expected to decrease problematic behavior; (2) incentives or reinforcing consequences that might be expected to increase appropriate behavior; and (3) preventive procedures or antecedent interventions that might be expected to pre-empt the development of problematic behavior. A behavioral procedure was scored as present if the review described agency use of that technique with a keyword (e.g., "token system") or a synonymous phrase (e.g., "program in which tokens and rewards are earned").

Five restrictive procedures or potentially reductive consequences were scored:

1. *Social disapproval* (e.g., administering verbal reprimands);
2. *Token or point fines* (removing tokens or points contingent on the performance of inappropriate behavior);
3. *Privilege removal* (temporarily removing privileges or demoting a youth's level contingent on the performance of inappropriate behavior);
4. *Restriction* (temporarily confining a youth to his bedroom or some other section of the group living area contingent on the performance of inappropriate behavior); and,
5. *"Timeout"* (temporary confinement within an empty room contingent on the performance of inappropriate behavior).

Four incentive or potentially reinforcing consequences were scored:

1. *Social reinforcement* (e.g., giving praise or other positive recognition for desired behavior);
2. *Token system* (dispensing tokens or some other substitute currency for desired behavior that could later be exchanged for material rewards);
3. *Point system* (using points or some other tally count for desired behavior that could later be redeemed for material rewards); and,
4. *Level system* (utilizing a program of tiered privileges to motivate improvements in behavior).

In addition to the programmatic consequences mentioned above, five antecedent interventions were also scored. Derived from research with developmentally disabled clients (Bailey & Pyles, 1989; Pyles & Bailey, 1990), these antecedent interventions could prevent the emergence of problem behavior by preempting or satisfying a need that might motivate aggressive, disruptive, self-injurious, or other aberrant behavior. Although these antecedent interventions are not often cited in the child welfare literature and are not mandated by state regulations, they are non-aversive and practical approaches to improving client behavior and the detailed program descriptions in the compliance reviews made it possible to reliably score the presence or absence of these items. The five antecedent interventions and potential preventive interventions scored were:

1. *Activity schedules* (setting regular times for activities of daily living as well as arranging varied social and recreational events);
2. *Environmental structure* (making room assignments and seating arrangements based on the compatibility of youth, monitoring level of crowding, ambient noise and temperature, and other conditions in the living environment that might favorably or adversely effect youths' behavior);
3. *Biological needs* (monitoring to ensure that youths' physiological needs were being met and that they were not affected by conditions such as hunger, thirst, pain, fatigue, physical illness, or medication side effects);
4. *Suitable demands* (adjusting assigned tasks to maximize their acceptability, considering factors such as difficulty of task, pace of work, and youth's preference for the activity); and,
5. *Redirection* (nonchalantly diverting youth from inappropriate to appropriate behavior through verbal or gestural prompts, or both).

Availability of Professional Staff. Since trained professionals are presumably best qualified to oversee the application of clinical interventions, research assistants also recorded the number of full-time "social workers" and "psychologists" employed at each agency. Reports did not always specify the educational background of the professionals in question (e.g., whether "social workers" held bachelors or masters degrees in social work); therefore, these were job titles rather than exact professional categories, and they presented an optimistic picture of professional expertise available on-site to oversee clinical procedures. Nevertheless, it is reasonable to assume that a positive correlation existed between the number of staff occupying professional job titles and the number of persons within the agency with a professional education.

Relationships between variables were investigated with query commands and logical "AND" functions of a database software. These functions calculated the joint occurrence of particular interventions, and the joint occurrence of particular interventions and types of staff.

For example, one query was used to sort out agencies that used "timeout," and a second query was performed on this subset of agencies to sort out those that also used point systems, or level systems, or both.

Interrater Reliability

Reliability checks were performed on the scoring of behavioral interventions, the aspect of data collection that required the greatest amount of interpretation by the observers. For 30% of the reviews, two research assistants independently read and scored the same reviews for the presence or absence of the 14 behavioral program components. Interrater reliability was computed with phi, a correlational coefficient appropriate for dichotomous data (Edwards, 1976). Only those categories with reliability that equaled or exceeded .75 were retained for subsequent study.

RESULTS

Interrater Reliability

Interrater reliability coefficients for the 14 behavioral programming components are displayed in Table 1. As shown in the table, of the behavior reduction procedures only privilege removal and "timeout" satisfied the reliability criterion with coefficients of .75 and .85, respectively. Of the positive reinforcement procedures, point and level systems met the criterion for subsequent analysis with reliability coefficients of .86 and 1.00, respectively. Of the antecedent interventions, redirection was the sole procedure mentioned in the program reviews and its reliability was .84.

Agency Usage of Behavioral Procedures

For official state programs reviews conducted during 1984-94, a total of 62% (126/204) of the audited agencies used one or more of the five behavioral interventions that this study was able to track reliably. The number and percentage of agencies using specific behavioral interventions are shown in the first column of Table 2. Only one antecedent intervention, redirection, was applied by a mere 22% of the reviewed agencies. Systematic use of consequences was more common, with roughly comparable usage of positive reinforcement and behavior reduction procedures in 38-52% of the agencies.

TABLE 1. Interrater Reliability for Behavioral Procedures (*phi*)

Reductive Consequences/Restrictive Procedures	
Social disapproval/reprimands	n.r.[a]
Token or point fines	.71
Privilege removal	.75
Restriction	.55
Confinement/timeout	.85
Reinforcing Consequences/Positive Incentives	
Social reinforcement	.71
Token system	.63
Point system	.86
Level system	1.00
Antecedent Interventions	
Activity schedules	n.r.
Environmental structure	n.r.
Biological state	n.r.
Demand characteristics	n.r.
Redirection	.84

[a]Not reported (n.r.) in agency compliance reviews.

TABLE 2. Substitute Care Agencies Using Behavioral Interventions and Professional Staff Available for Supervision

Procedure	No. of Agencies	No. with Full-time "Social Worker"	No. with Full-time "Psychologist"
Redirection	28 (22%)[a]	10 (36%)[b]	1 (4%)[b]
Point System	49 (38%)	19 (39%)	6 (12%)
Level System	61 (48%)	13 (21%)	5 (8%)
Privilege Removal	48 (38%)	13 (27%)	5 (10%)
"Timeout"	67 (52%)	21 (31%)	5 (7%)

[a] Percentages in the first column based on n = 126 (number of agencies reporting use of at least one behavioral intervention).
[b] Percentages in the second and third columns based on the number reported in the first column (number of agencies reporting use of that particular procedure).

Availability of Professional Staff

Results showed that the numbers of professional "social workers" and "psychologists" employed by the audited agencies were quite small. The number and percentage of agencies reporting employment of at least one full-time "social worker" or "psychologist" (separated according to type of behavioral interventions utilized by the agency) are displayed in the second and third columns of Table 2. The percentage of agencies using behavioral procedures that identified a full-time "social worker" as being a member of their staff ranged from 21-39%. A substantially smaller number proportion of agencies reported having a full-time "psychologist" employed at their agency with percentages ranging from only 4-12%.

Reinforcement and Behavior Reduction Procedures

Data on the joint usage of positive reinforcement and behavior reduction procedures are displayed in Table 3. Of the 48 agencies that reported applying privilege removal 31% reported using point or level systems, 41% reported using both point and level systems, and 27% reported using neither point nor level systems. Joint usage of positive reinforcement and behavior reduction procedures was lower for the more restrictive procedure of "timeout." Of the 67 agencies that reported applying "timeout" only 19% reported using point or level systems, 16% repoted using both point and level systems, and 64% reported using neither point nor level systems.

A possible relationship between agencies' usage of point and level systems and "timeout" was evaluated by computing a phi coefficient

TABLE 3. Use of Reinforcement and Behavior Reduction Procedures in State-Funded Agencies

Reinforcement Procedures	Behavior Reduction Procedures	
	Privilege Removal (n = 48)	"Timeout" (n = 67)
Point System	2% (1) [a]	6% (4)
Level System	29% (14)	13% (9)
Point and Level Systems	41% (20)	16% (11)
None	27% (13)	64% (43)

[a]Figure in parentheses is the number of agencies reporting usage of the procedure.

and a chi-square test of independence on this data. Due to the low frequency of programs using only point systems or only level systems, these categories were combined with the point and level system category. A phi coefficient quantifying the relationship between usage of reinforcement procedures (i.e., use of point, level, or point and level systems vs. no use of these procedures) and type of behavior reduction procedure (i.e., privilege removal vs. "timeout") revealed a negative correlation of phi = –.34. A test of independence yielded an obtained chi square of 15.41, (df = 1), indicating a statistically significant relationship (p < .0001). These data indicate agencies that applied timeout were significantly less likely to utilize any form of reinforcement procedure.

DISCUSSION

This study of one state's substitute care facilities found that a relatively large proportion of state-funded facilities use behavioral procedures to manage youths' behavioral and conduct problems. However, the types of interventions applied, the lack of coordination between procedures used, and the number of professionals available to supervise their use give cause for concern. First, agencies rarely used antecedent behavioral interventions that could preempt or prevent behavior disturbances. In other words, simple techniques that could obviate the need for restrictive procedures, such as minimizing irritating stimuli or taking individual preferences into account, were not widely incorporated in therapeutic residential programs.

Second, positive reinforcement, response cost, and "timeout" procedures often were not applied together in a logically or theoretically sound manner. A majority of audited agencies that reported using privilege removal also employed point or level systems, or both; however, nearly a third of the agencies using privilege removal had neither point nor level systems. The data indicate that the latter third of these agencies had programs in which formal mechanisms existed for withdrawing privileges and desired objects for inappropriate behavior, but no parallel mechanisms that allowed youth to earn privileges or rewards for appropriate behavior. Agency programs may not actually have been structured like this, and some positive incentives may have been present in these settings. Nonetheless, important educative and motivational functions of positive reinforcement were not reflected in the formal program of these agencies. Such programs contradict basic behavioral principles which aim to teach adaptive skills and prosocial responses by providing positive consequences following the desired behavior.

Programmatic errors in the use of "timeout" were even more serious than those found with the use of privilege removal. Nearly two-thirds of the agencies that reported using this more restrictive procedure had neither a point nor a level system in place. So, once again, agency programs were structured to discourage inappropriate behavior by restricting access to desired activities and objects following its occurrence; but, they did not promote appropriate behavior by dispensing privileges or positive rewards following its occurrence. This error may have degraded the intervention to the point where it was not even nominally effective. Behavioral research has shown that placing clients in "timeout" following problem behavior is unlikely to decrease that behavior unless the "timein" situation is more reinforcing than the "timeout" situation (Cooper, Heron, & Heward, 2006; Solnick, Rincover, & Peterson, 1977). Use of "timeout" when the "timein" situation does not have a relatively higher reinforcing value may actually increase rather than decrease problem behavior. Unfortunately, many substitute care programs seemed to be assembled without regard for the amount of positive reinforcement in the milieu, as evidenced in the large number of programs that did not systematically provide privileges, material items, or other positive reinforcement for desired behavior. These agencies appeared to use "timeout" programs in a punitive manner for purposes of group control, but applied in a technically improper manner this procedure may have been ineffective or even counter-therapeutic.

Shortage of properly trained staff is one probable factor contributing to the faulty application of behavioral procedures noted in this study. Masters-level social workers and doctoral-level psychologists, professionals who would have the best likelihood of taking graduate-level courses in this methodology, were scarce in these agencies. It should be noted, however, that formal education in social work or psychology would not necessarily involve study of behavioral principles and methods. Therefore, even professional staff with appropriate degrees might not have received specialized training in learning theory, behavioral interventions, and single-case research methodology needed to select and evaluate suitable treatments. The present data suggest that behavioral procedures applied in these state agencies are most likely implemented and overseen by paraprofessionals, or persons with bachelor's degrees at best. This is especially problematic for behavioral interventions because they are complex and their correct application can be counter-intuitive.

One limitation of the present results is that it was based on information reported by agency staff. Descriptions of behavioral interventions given in agency documents did not guarantee that these procedures were actually implemented on residential units or that they were implemented properly. Derived primarily from written reports, this study was unable to accurately gauge the integrity of behavioral programs. Conversely, behavioral interventions that were not described in agency documents or that raters were unable to score reliably might still have been applied with youth in these facilities. This study only assessed the *reported* presence or absence of behavioral procedures and whether the relationships between these reported procedures were theoretically sound. To accurately assess agency programs, written program descriptions must be validated by direct observations of staff/client interactions to show the actual performance of approved procedures (DeRoos & Pinkston, 1997; Ivancic et al., 1981; Schinke & Wong, 1977).

Results of the present study indicate that regulatory prohibitions may protect clients from the most hazardous or objectionable behavior management procedures, but not provide technically sound or effective treatment. This state's regulations established minimum standards for behavior management practices, but left much to be desired in terms of facilitating the development of humane, state-of-the-art behavioral interventions. Future research is needed to determine whether the present results are representative of conditions in substitute care facilities in other states and whether the quality of behavioral programming has improved in recent years.

REFERENCES

Bailey, J. S., & Pyles, D. A. M. (1989). Behavioral diagnostics. *Monographs of the American Association on Mental Retardation, 12*, 85-106.

Burns, B. J., Phillips, S. D., Wagner, H. R., Barth, R. P., Kolko, D. J., Campbell, Y., & Landsverk, J. (2004). Mental health need and access to mental health services by youths involved with child welfare: A national survey. *Journal of the Academy of Child and Adolescent Psychiatry, 43*(8), 960-970.

Chamberlain, P., & Moore, K. (1998). Models of community treatment for serious juvenile offenders. In J. Crane (Ed.), *Social programs that work* (pp. 258-276). New York, NY: Russell Sage Foundation.

Cooper, J. O., Heron, T. E., & Heward, W. L. (2006). *Applied behavior analysis* (2nd ed.). Upper Saddle River, NJ: Prentice Hall.

DeRoos, Y. S., & Pinkston, E. M. (1997). Training adult-day-care staff. In D. M. Baer & E. M. Pinkston (Eds.), *Environment and behavior* (pp. 249-257). Boulder, CO: Westview Press.

Edwards, A. L. (1976). *An introduction to linear regression and correlation.* San Francisco, CA: W. H. Freeman and Company.

Foltz, R. (2004). The efficacy of residential treatment: An overview of the evidence. *Residential Treatment for Children & Youth, 22*(2), 1-19.

Hurley, K. D., Ingram, S., Czyz, J. D., Juliano, N., & Wilson, E. (2006). Treatment for youth in short-term care facilities: The impact of a comprehensive behavior management intervention. *Journal of Child and Family Studies, 15*(5), 617-632.

Ivancic, M. T., Reid, D. H., Iwata, B. A., Faw, G. D., & Page, T. J. (1981). Evaluating a supervision program for developing and maintaining therapeutic staff-resident interactions during institutional care routines. *Journal of Applied Behavior Analysis, 14*(1), 95-107.

Lietz, C. A. (2004). Resiliency based social learning: A strengths based approach to residential treatment. *Residential Treatment for Children & Youth, 22*(2), 21-36.

Pyles, D. A. M., & Bailey, J. S. (1990). Diagnosing severe behavior problems. In A. C. Repp & N. N. Singh (Eds.), *Perspectives on the use of nonaversive and aversive interventions for persons with developmental disabilities* (pp. 381-401). Sycamore, IL: Sycamore Publishing Company.

Murray, L., & Sefchik, G. (1992). Regulating behavior management practices in residential treatment facilities. *Children and Youth Services Review, 14*(6), 519-539.

Nabors, L., Sumajin, I., Zins, J., Rofey, D., Berberich, D., Brown, S., & Weist, M. (2003). Evaluation of an intervention for children experiencing homelessness. *Child and Youth Care Forum, 32*(4), 211-227.

Schinke, S. P., & Wong, S. E. (1977). Evaluation of staff training in group homes for retarded persons. *American Journal of Mental Deficiency, 82*(2), 130-136.

Solnick, J. V., Rincover, A., & Peterson, C. R. (1977). Some determinants of the reinforcing and punishing effects of timeout. *Journal of Applied Behavior Analysis, 10*(3), 415-424.

Wong, S. E. (1999). Treatment of antisocial behavior in adolescent inpatients: Behavioral outcomes and clien satisfaction. *Research on Social Work Practice, 9*(1), 25-44.

Wong, S. E. (in press). Operant learning theory. In K. M. Sowers, C. N. Dulmus, & B. A. Thyer (Eds.), *Comprehensive handbook of social work and social welfare: Vol. 2. Human behavior in the social environment.* New York: John Wiley and Sons.

Continuity of Care and Outcomes in Residential Care:
A Comparison of Two Care Giving Models

Loring Jones, DSW

INTRODUCTION

In residential care the primary responsibility for treatment of residents resides with professionals who usually have advanced degrees that qualify them to diagnose and treat problems. The care giving staff (CGS) in residential care has less training, authority, and prestige than the professional staff. CGS do not diagnosis or provide treatment in the formal sense, but they are expected to establish relationships with youth that will help the residents use the treatment services of the facility. CGS, such as child care workers and house parents, provide the bulk of contact with residents, and are responsible for supervising that period of the resident's day outside of diagnosis and treatment (Bettelheim & Sanders, 1979; Leichtman, 2006). Even if they do not provide treatment CCG workers are regarded as paraprofessional members of a treatment team. An assumption of residential treatment is that all interactions have a potential to be part of the therapeutic treatment. Data from youth gathered both during and post residential placement suggest that the relationship with the care giving staff were among the most important and meaningful component of their residential experiences (Anglin, 2004; Devine, 2004; Smith, McKay, & Chakrabrat, 2004). Therefore, CGS in residential care are regarded as crucial parts of the intervention program. Despite the importance of CGS, not much is known about how they contribute to the therapeutic milieu and treatment outcomes (Little, Kohm, & Thompson, 2005; Moses, 2001).

This paper reports on a research study that examined differences in two residential care-giving models (houseparent vs. child care worker) in providing continuity of care for youth, and examines how this continuity affects selected outcomes. An aspect of residential life that is crucial for youth is the continuity that they experience in care giving. Youth in care have a history that often includes maltreatment, and they have not experienced the consistency in parenting necessary to develop trust and security that is the foundation for subsequent healthy relationships (Barth, Courtney, Berrick, & Albert, 1994). Out-of-home care is also a disruptive and potentially traumatic experience for children unable to remain with their biological parents. Residential care is expected to partially make up for these deficits.

CGS is expected to help create and maintain a safe and predictable environment for youth (Szajnberg, 1985) that has the flexibility to adapt to the needs of individual youth (Feist, Slowiak, & Colligan, 1985). They are supposed to make use of every day events to accomplish therapeutic goals (Fitzgerald, 1995).

The role set of the CGS is complex and lengthy. Caregivers are expected act as surrogate parents (e, g, feeding, attending to youth hygiene, helping with homework, providing discipline, developing independent living skills), provide intervention (e.g., counseling, crisis intervention, life space interviews, facilitate the use of services), act as a custodian (assure safety, maintaining the daily routine), and attend to the social needs of the child (e.g., take on outings, engage in recreation, etc.) (Moses, 2001).

From a practice perspective, the significance of questions about choice of a care taking model have to do with the attachment issues between caretaker and the child, the commitment of caregivers to youth, and the stability of the residential environment. Wahler (1994) has described a concept that he called social continuity that is essential for work with children and youth. Continuity is defined as interactions by caretakers directed at youth that are predictable, appropriate, and occur over an extended period time. This pattern of interaction is necessary for the youth to believe that they have relationships on which they can depend and anticipate. Continuity of care giving is essential for youth who have a history of disrupted relationships with families, experience with multiple placements, and who for one reason or other have many different transitory relationships with helping professionals.

Glisson and Hemmelgarn (1998) view continuity as an essential component of the client/worker relationship because clients were more likely to view workers with whom they had continual relationships as more responsive and available than they viewed workers with whom the relationship was of a briefer duration. This perception of responsiveness and availability was associated with improved psychosocial functioning.

The literature on foster youth overwhelmingly supports the notion that frequent change of placement is a significant risk to a youth's psychosocial development (Barth, Courtney, Berrick, & Albert, 1994; Newton, Litronick, & Landsverk, 2000; Smith, Stormshack, Chamberlain, & Whaley, 2001). This risk operates largely through the absence of a consistent caregiver with whom the youth can develop a caring relationship. What has not been investigated is whether children who are in stable placements, but who have frequent change of caregivers, are exposed to the same developmental risks. Based on the literature, one could hypothesize that a lack of continuity in caregiving, even without placement change, can pose a risk for youth.

This paper describes how care giving models provide continuity for youth in residential care. The houseparent model and child care worker model are the main caregiving models for youth in residential care. Differences between these models are summarized in Table 1.

TABLE 1. Comparison of Care Giving Models

Characteristics	Biological Parents	House Parents	Child Care Workers
Physical environment	Care in Own home	Cottage system	Agency house in the community or Institution
# of Youth in care	1-5+	8-10	8-100+
Time element	Full-time and continuous across life cycle	Full-time while in care, some respite	Shift work
Intensity of care	Familial care	Family like environment	Staff care with elements of therapeutic care
Respite	Low	Medium	High
Style of care	Intimate	Intimate to informal	Informal to formal
Living Arrangements of Caretaker	Usually in a family home	Live on site with child	Lives off site
Caretaker Compensation	Unpaid	Better pay than child care	Low pay
Economic costs	Assumed less expensive than out-of-home care	More expensive than child care workers	Less expensive than house parents

Adapted from Anglin (2002A).

Houseparent Model

One example of the house parent model is the Boy's Town treatment approach. The site where data were gathered for this study originally utilized the Boy's Town approach when it began operations. This model assumes that a "family like" environment is needed in residential care, and can be best maintained by live-in workers referred to as house parents. House parents are supposed to help create a "family like" environment that would more closely resemble the home than one would find in a childcare model, and thus project a degree of normality into the artificial environment of the group home. House parents in theory provide an intimate and nurturing environment that gives a youth a sense of belonging and stability, and helps them utilize the intervention program. The sense of nurturance also allows the youth to learn how to be in a family and work through some of the trauma that comes from the loss of their biological family (Daly, Scmidt, & Spellman, 1998; Terpestra, 1998; U.S. Government Accounting Office, 1994).

This model utilizes a teaching family headed by a married couple acting as surrogate parents. These parents participate in such activities as shopping with youth, taking them to medical appointments, attending school functions, and helping them with their homework. The youth have household responsibilities such as cleaning their rooms and preparing meals, and thus have opportunities to learn independent living skills. The assumption of the model is that house parents would be available to the youth for five full days a week, but with weekend relief from other staff (Daly et al., 1998).

Critics of the house parent model view it as unrealistic and competitive with the biological family. Anglin (2002B, 2004) asserted that many youth from intact families, who were living in residential care, viewed the attempts to imitate families unfavorably, and these efforts could cause a youth to be confused about the identity of their own family. Anglin (2002B) also suggests youth benefited from having a diverse child care staff comprised of many different adults with whom the youth could develop a variety of relationships.

Anglin's view is not universally held. Devine (2004) reported that youth in residential care who were in family style living arrangements reported a critical sense of belonging that they had not experienced in their own families. Moore and colleagues (1998) in describing a residential program that utilized Attachment Theory in its intervention emphasized limiting the number the number of staff members with whom a youth interacts in order to intensify those relationships. This intensity would make it more likely that youth would form attachment relationships with staff.

The unrealistic aspects of considering the house parent model are several. The house parent does not provide continuity across the life cycle that biological parents give, and the job title may contain expectations of what children can expect from the relationship to the caregiver that cannot be met. For example, the house parent's scope of decision-making is much narrower than one would expect in a biological family. Residential administrators, or the social workers from the placing agency, and not the house parents, have the final decision about what happens to the youth.

Child Care Workers

The child care worker model uses staff to provide supervision of children or youth in rotating shifts. Child care workers engage primarily in the behavioral management of the residents, and often help carry out specific intervention programs. They are less likely to engage in household or independent living skills training activities than are house parents (Pecora & Gingerich, 1981). For example, they might not work a shift where they would have an opportunity to engage in meal preparation activities with youth.

Crucial distinctions between the models are that the child care worker does not reside in the cottage, works on shifts, and may rotate among residential units. Anglin (2002A) regards the ability to get away from the facility as vital to the worker because they have time to rejuvenate. This respite is necessary due to the stressful nature of the job.

Child care workers tend to be younger than house parents, poorly paid, with a high tendency toward turnover (Berrick, 1993). Child care workers at the current study site reported to the researcher that they view their role as a "counselor" and "friend" rather than as a surrogate parent. They are not just expected to be a custodian of their charges, but they are expected to make judgments about behavior and intervene appropriately. The facility where this research was conducted required child care workers to have a Bachelor's degree or commensurate work experience prior to hiring which is a common requirement for child care workers. Anglin (2002A) notes the importance of an undergraduate degree in the social or behavioral sciences for providing child care workers with the knowledge to understand and cope with youth who have multiple problems.

High turnover among child care workers has been noted as a factor that limits the effectiveness of residential programs, and hinders the attachment of youth to staff (Berrick, 1993; Ross, 1983). Low pay, lack of benefits, low status, inconvenient work shifts, and a lack of career ladders may discourage workers from making a long term commitment to child care work. High turnover may mean residential facilities are often hiring inexperienced workers just to keep programs fully staffed (Ross, 1983).

THE CONTEXT OF THE STUDY

The residential program where this study was conducted opened in October 2001 and was meant to serve as an innovative long-term placement option for adolescent foster youth who had no other placement options, and who were not likely to return to their biological families. The program was intended to provide a stable home and a comprehensive educational program in preparation for emancipation from the foster care system.

The designers of the program wished to maintain a "family like" environment, and this intent was directly expressed in the architectural layout and original staffing of the residential unit. The residential physical environment was designed as a cottage system with a capacity of up to eight students per cottage unit. Each cottage contains a family room, dining room, kitchen, bedrooms for youth, and a small apartment for house parents. The apartment enables the house parents to be on site for extended periods. Living on site is a crucial and distinctive feature of the model. The family environment was to be nested within the intervention program staffed by a variety of professionals.

The residential program was initially designed to use the house parent model. Shortly after the facility began operation the residential contractor began to slowly shift to the child care model. The contractor found it difficult to implement the parent model primarily due to costs. State and federal labor laws required that employees working more than 40 hours receive overtime pay. The house parent model assumes the caregiver is available outside of the traditional workday, and the contractor interpreted state law to mean that this availability required additional compensation. Even without overtime the house parents were considerably more expensive than child care workers (Short, 1980; Berrick, 1993). At the study site each house parent received a $25,000 yearly salary. Child care workers were hourly employees who earned about $16,600 a year if employed full time. All of the house parents were full time employees, but only a portion of the child care workers were full time, and thus many child care workers did not receive benefits. When house parents were off duty child care workers provided supervision, but as much as possible the work schedules for house parents were arranged so as to maximize contact with the residents. For example, house parents were on duty before and after school, and off duty when youth were sleeping.

The facility eventually operated on a hybrid model with some cottages having house parents, and others having child care workers. At intake youth were assigned to cottages by a mixture of bed availability, and clinical judgment. The clinical judgment piece consisted of staff making an assessment about which cottage was the "best fit" for a youth. "Fit" entailed determining how the youth's age, personality, and behavioral profile might blend in with the caretakers and residents living in the unit. This author saw no evidence that youth were assigned a residence based on a caretaker models ability to manage behavioral problems. As a matter of fact the residential contractor was skeptical that the house parent model offered any advantages over child care workers.

The author was conducting an evaluation of the residential program that included data collection from youth and caretakers. It was the belief of the researcher that the change in care giving models provided a unique opportunity to study these care giving models in the same context. Examining these models at the same facility would control for some of the confounding variables that might result from study of these forms of caregiving in different settings.

METHOD

The purposes of this research were to examine whether a care giving model was associated with continuity of care, and whether continuity had an effect on selected outcomes such as the exhibition of behavior problems, the acquisition of independent living skills, and the youth's satisfaction with the quality of their life. It was hypothesized that youth who had house parents would experience more continuity than youth with child care workers. Continuity was defined as continual contact with the same primary caregiver. It was further hypothesized that youth experiencing higher levels of continuity would have better outcomes than youth experiencing lower levels of continuity. Better outcomes meant that the youth would experience fewer behavioral problems, exhibit more independent living skills, and would be more satisfied with their quality of life than youth with poorer outcomes.

Sample and Data Collection

Case files of all 290 residents who entered the residence from its opening in October of 2001 through the summer of 2005. Data were abstracted from the records of these youth through June of 2006. These data were used to gauge the continuity of care giving. Interview data was available on the first eighty-seven residents to the facility who had been in residence for six months. Graduate level research assistants who were trained in the use of the instrument interviewed youth at the entrance into the residential placement (baseline), and again four months later. Care takers were interviewed at a two month lag to the youth interviews. This lag to baseline youth interviews was meant to ensure that they had observed the youth over a sufficient enough amount of time in order to accurately describe their adjustment to placement. The purpose of the second interview was to assess youth progress in the program.

Study Domains and Measures

The data for examining continuity were drawn from the "Student Home Assignment" sheet generated monthly by residential staff. This document lists whether a cottage had house parents or child care workers assigned to it, and provides a listing of the residents of the cottage. We began by determining the kind of caregivers a youth experienced. The type of caregiver a youth had was categorized for month the youth was in residence. A variable was created that gave a ratio for each youth of the percentage of time they had a house parent.

The *degree of continuity* was determined by the number of months the youth had the same caretaker regardless of whether they had house parents or child care workers. This variable reflected the longest relationship they had with a single caretaker while in residence, and was a ratio of the number of months in residence that the youth had that caretaker as their primary caregiver. Computing this variable was fairly simple for house parents, but for the child care worker a number of assumptions had to be made. Many child care workers cycled through the cottages including the house parent staffed cottages. In a house parent cottage we assumed that the most significant relationship that youth had would be with the parent. Cottages staffed by child care workers had a worker designated as the lead worker. The lead worker was treated as a house parent, and as the youth's primary caregiver. The researchers assumed if the youth had the same lead worker month to month they were experiencing continuous care in the cottage.

The second means to establish continuity was to determine how many caregiver changes (called *Turnover* in the Tables) in house parents and lead child care workers a youth experienced. Fewer changes meant that the youth had more continuity. Changes in child care workers were counted if the person designated as the lead worker left the cottage. Because youth were in the facility for different period of times we needed to standardize this variable by transforming it into a measure of the likelihood that in any given month of residence the youth would experience a change of caretakers. The number of caretaker changes a child experienced was divided by the number of months in residence.

Youth movement through the cottages was also tracked. A variable was created that measured whether a youth moved or not during their first six months of residence (called *Move* in the analysis). The purpose of this variable was to assess if this change in living environment might have the same negative affects that have been demonstrated with placement change. Twenty-four months of data were available for the continuity variables. It was hypothesized that youth who had house parents would experience more continuity, and fewer changes of caretakers than youth with child care workers.

The following were data gathered in interviews with the youth and caretaker.

Annual Client Evaluation (ACE) developed by Wilson and Conroy (1999) to assess foster youth's satisfaction with their living arrangements and the overall quality of their life. The instrument contains items on the youth's satisfaction with various aspects of their lives and services (health, school, peers, recreation, clothes, comfort, perception of safety, food, bedroom or private space, feeling loved, and happiness), the self-perceived quality of life before and during placement, the youth's relationship with staff, and other youth living with them. The reliability of the ACE was tested with a test-retest method with 250 foster children in Illinois. The overall rating on most items was between 86% and 100%.

Youth in the current sample were asked at baseline to comment on their satisfaction with their previous placement. Residents provided an assessment of their satisfaction with the current placement 4 months later. It was hypothesized that youth with houseparent would show more satisfaction with the quality of their life than youth with child care workers. This scale showed high reliability with the current sample (alpha = .90).

House parents and lead child care workers completed the *Child Behavior Checklist–11 to 18 version* (CBCL) at baseline but at the lag described earlier. The CBCL instruments measure the youth's behavioral, emotional, and social competencies and problems (total problems, externalizing and internalizing syndromes) (Achenbach, 1991). The CBCL demonstrated excellent reliability in the current study (alpha = .89). This measure is widely used in studies of children's mental health and provides the information about the behavioral adjustment of the youth. It was hypothesized that youth with house parents, and/or greater continuity of care, would express fewer behavioral problems than youth with child care workers and/or who had had lesser amounts of continuity of care. Caretakers completed a second CBCL for the resident about 6 months after the youth entered the facility.

The *Ansel-Casey Life Skills Assessment-Short Version* (ACLSA) was developed by the Casey Family Program as a means of assessing foster youth's readiness for independent living (Casey Family Program, 1998). Caretakers completed this version twice in the same time frame as the CBCL. This instrument measures the needs and competencies of youth in the following independent living skills (ILS) areas; social development, knowledge about sex and pregnancy, money management, and daily living skills. The alpha coefficient was .96. It was hypothesized that youth with house parents would demonstrate more acquisition of ILS than youth with child care workers.

FINDINGS

Describing the Residents

Demographic characteristics of the sample are shown in Table 2. Male and female students are compared at entrance. Almost 60% of the students were 15 to 16 years old. More girls than boys were in residence. No other statistically significant differences by gender on age, race/ethnicity, or grade level were found. About two-thirds of the students were of Caucasian or African-American race/ethnicity. Twenty-one percent of students were Hispanic. Boys had received child protective services for a significantly longer period time and had more placements than girls. These frequent placement changes are one reason why the researcher believes continuity of caregiving is important for this group.

Two overall patterns emerge from inspection of this Table. At intake the adult caretakers report behavioral problems for a much larger proportion of students than would be expected from the general population. In the general population, approximately 5% to 10% of youth would be in the borderline/clinical range on these measures. Adult caretakers report problems that would classify about one-third of the student in this borderline/clinical range on the "Total Behavior Problems" and "Externalizing Behavior Problems" scales. The caretakers said that slightly less than 20% of students have scores on the "Internalizing Behavior Problems" scale that would place them in the borderline/clinical range. Other studies of children in care that utilize the CBCL found results comparable to the current findings. Overall, the youth seem representative of children in care (Armsden, Pecora, Payne, & Szatkiewicz, 1999).

The second pattern seen in the data is that female students were exhibiting higher levels of behavior problems than male students. Caretakers reported significantly more problems on all three subscales of the CBCL for girls than they did for boys.

TABLE 2. Description of Students at Entrance to the Residential Program

Domain/Variable	Male Students N = 128	Female Students n = 162	All Students n = 290
Demographic Characteristics			
Age:*			
12	11.1%	2.4%	6.4%
13-14	31.9%	23.5%	27.4%
15-16	48.6%	58.8%	54.1%
17-18	8.3%	15.3%	12.1%
Gender:**			
Male	100.0%		45.9%
Female		100.0%	54.1%
Race/Ethnicity:			
Caucasian	33.3%	37.6%	35.7%
African-American	33.3%	31.8%	32.5%
Hispanic	22.2%	20.0%	21.0%
Asian/Pacific Islander	0.0%	5.9%	3.2%
Native American	9.7%	3.5%	6.4%
Bi-Racial	1.4%	1.2%	1.3%
	Male Students N = 66	**Female Students n = 73**	**All Students n = 139**
Caretaker Report of Problem Behaviors (CBCL)			
Total Behavior Problems Within Borderline/Clinical Range**	22.7%	41.1%	32.4%
Externalizing Behavior Problems Within Borderline/Clinical Range*	27.3%	38.4%	33.1%
Internalizing Behavior Problems Within Borderline/Clinical range	10.6%	28.8%	19.3%
	N = 120	**N = 155**	**N = 275**
Placement Stability	**Mean (sd)**	**Mean (sd)**	**Mean (sd)**
MEAN # OF PLACEMENTS***	7.34 (5.18)	7.04(4.76)	7.17 (4.94)
Mean # of Year in Child Protective Services Prior to the Current Placement ***	6.71(4.27)	5.71(4.24)	6.15(4.27)

* Differences between groups (male and female) were statistically significant at the p < .05 level.
**Differences between groups (male and female) were statistically significant at the p < .01 level.
+Differences from 100% due to rounding error.

Continuity of Care

Table 3 describes residents' experience with the care giving models, continuity, and movement within the residential setting. Pearson's r is used to test relationships. The continuity variables describe up to 24 months of the youth's experience at the residence. The variables from the interview data show the youth's experience after 4 to 6 months at the facility. As hypothesized youth who had house parents had more continuous contact with the same care giver ($r = .656$, $p < .0001$), and youth with house parents experienced fewer changes of caretakers (called Turnover in Table 3, $r = -.780$, $p < .0001$). The Turnover coefficient suggests that house parents were less likely to leave the cottage than were child care workers. Youth, who had more contact with child care workers than house parents, had more internal behavioral problems ($r = -.298$, $p < .0001$) and total problems ($r = -.232$, $p < .05$) than did youth living in house parent staffed cottages. However, youth with child care workers

TABLE 3. Correlation Matrix: The Impact of Care Giver Type at the Second Interview 2

	HP	Continuity	TO	Move	CBCL-I	CBCL-E	CBCL-TP
Houseparent (HP) n = 290	—						
Continuity n = 290	.656***	—					
Turnover (TO) n = 290	−.780***	−.710***	—				
Move (n = 290)	.030	−.064	.016	—			
CBCL-I (n = 87)	−298**	−344***	−390***	.039	—		
CBCL-E (n = 87)	−.117	−.241*	−.239*	−.072	.611***	—	
CBCL-TP (n = 87)	−.232*	−.305**	−.340***	−.037	.845***	.851***	—
ACE (n = 87)	−.175+	−.076	.030	−.073	−.100	−.047	−.037
ACLSA (n = 87)	.017	.030	.010	−.181+	−.008	.090	.042

a. Tested with Pearson's r.
b. CBCL-I=Internalization problems.
c. CBCL-E=Externalization problems.
d. CBCL-TP= Total problems.
***p <. 0001, **p < .001, *p < .05, +p < .10.

appeared to be more satisfied with their quality of life (ACE, $r = -.175$, $p < .099$) than youth with house parents, but this difference only approached significance.

Forty-three youth (36.1%) moved in their first four months of residence. Staff reported that youth were more likely to move in the first few months of residence as the care givers became aware of the youth's specific needs, and might decide another cottage was a better fit for the youth. Fifty-six percent of the youth who moved said they were at least somewhat dissatisfied with their initial cottage, and 54% of these residents said they were at least somewhat satisfied with the change. Reasons given by CGS for changing a youth's cottage were: staff change in the cottage necessitated moving the youth (27.5%), youth had problems with other cottage residents (22.5%), staff thought another cottage would suit the youth better (20%), youth had problems with caregivers (15%), no reason given by staff (10%), and the youth wanted a change (5%). A youth movement to a new cottage was not significantly associated with any of the outcome variables, but was near a significant association with the acquisition of ILS ($r = -.181, p < .08$). The direction of the coefficient indicates that a youth's change of cottage was associated with fewer ILS skills as measured by the Ansel Casey.

Youth who reported more total problems had less continuous contact with their primary caregiver than those youth with more continuous contact. The house parent ratio was significantly associated with expressing both fewer internalizing difficulties ($r = -.298, p < .001$) and total problems ($r = -.232, p < .05$). The direction of the coefficients suggests youth who had more contact with house parents had fewer problems.

Testing the hypotheses that house parents and/or continuity reduced behavioral problems, and were associated with greater life satisfaction, required a longitudinal test since the correlational data only provided data about associations. A dichotomous variable was created out of the house parent variable in order to accomplish this test. Youth who had a house parent at least 86% of the time, and had a house parent complete their CBCL were coded in the house parent category. Youth not meeting this definition were coded as having a child care worker. These youth had child care workers 14% to 78% of the time, but almost all of these residents had child care workers as their current primary care giver. This child care worker completed the second CBCL. These two groups were compared using the independent t-test. Results are reported in Table 4.

No differences were found between groups on the CBCL's and Quality of Life (ACE) measure at baseline, but at the second measure youth

TABLE 4. Differences in Key Measures Between Baseline and Follow-Up

Measure	Baseline			Follow-up		
	House Parent (n = 27)	Child Care Worker (n = 60)		House Parent (n = 27)	Child Care Worker (n = 60)	
	Mean (sd)	Mean (sd)	P-Value	Mean (sd)	Mean (sd)	P-Value
CBCL-I	46.52 (12.7)	48.98 (11.6)	.379	44.07 (11.2)	50.86 (13.7)	.005
CBCL-E	50.52 (12.5)	53.24 (14.5)	.403	50.96 (11.7)	54.37 (14.9)	.297
CBCL-P	47.37 (14.4)	50.86 (13.7)	.332	46.81 (11.6)	53.07 (14.6)	.036
ACE	41.42 (8.6)	40.05 (7.9)	NS	46.35 (8.9)	49.54 (7.9)	.108

who had more contact with house parents had fewer internalizing problems, and did not express as many total problems than youth with child care workers. Table 5 is a report of the final test of the hypotheses on continuity and outcomes. As reported in Table 2, females had significantly more behavioral problems at baseline. In order to control for the effect of gender a series of regressions containing the continuity measures and gender as independent variables were run with the CBCL subscales dependent. This series needs to be completed because the continuity variables were to highly correlated with one another to be in the same regression model.

The results indicate that having a house parent is no longer significant with the dependent variables when controlled for by gender, but house parents still shows a near significant association with the CBCL-Internalization scale (Beta = −.210, $p < .051$), but gender show a stronger association with that scale (Beta = −.274, $p < .011$). Continuity is significant with two CBCL scales, internalization and total problems, and near significant with the CBCL-external scale, even when gender is used as a control. The direction of the coefficients suggests fewer behavioral problems are associated house parents and/or high levels of continuity. A change of caretakers (Turnover) is no longer significant with any of the behavioral measures, but remains near significant with two scales, the Internalization and Total Problems scales. The Beta suggests that more change of caretakers is associated with more behavioral problems.

Six empirical generalizations emerge from the data: (1) Youth with house parents experience more continuity in care giving than those youth with child care workers. (2) House parents were less likely to turnover than child care workers. (3) Continuity of care was significantly associated

TABLE 5. Testing the Hypotheses in Multiple Regression

Dependent: CBCL–Internalization

Independent Variables	Beta	Standard Error	P-Value
Gender	−.274	2.592	.011
House Parent Ratio	−.210	7.49	.051

1 = male, 0 = female
R square = .156
Dependent: CBCLI–nternalization

Independent Variables	Beta	Standard Error	P-Value
Gender	−.267	2.51	.011
Continuity	−.270	5.53	.010

R square = .184
Dependent: CBCL–Internalization

Independent Variables	Beta	Standard Error	P-Value
Gender	−301	21.4	.006
Turnover	.219	2.6	.045

R square = .155
Dependent: CBCL–Total Problems

Independent Variables	Beta	Standard Error	P-Value
Gender	−.255	2.91	.017
Continuity	−.235	6.42	.027

R Square = .153
Dependent: CBCL–Externalization

Independent Variables	Beta	Standard Error	P-Value
Gender	−.131	2.059	.235
Continuity	−.205	6.729	.065

R Square= .074
Dependent: CBCL–Externalization

Independent Variables	Beta	Standard Error	P-Value
Gender	−.222	26.11	.057
Turnover	−.097	3.27	.403

R square= .076

with a reduction in internalization and total problems. (4) House parents were associated with a reduction in behavioral problems, but only at a near significant level when gender was used as a control variable. (5) A change of caretakers was associated with an increase in behavioral problems. (6) A youth change in cottages did not demonstrate any of the negative affects on behavior associated with placement change.

STUDY LIMITATIONS

Findings of the current study should be interpreted in the context of the limitations of the research. These limitations are: (1) the small sample size affects the ability to demonstrate statistically significant relationships, (2) the sample was drawn from a single site which limits the ability to generalize, (3) data in Table 3 are cross-sectional, therefore we cannot infer causality from that table, (4) youth were not randomly assigned to cottages so a selection bias that was not apparent to the researcher could have been operating, and (5) more data was available from the file abstraction portion than the interview portion. This unevenness occurred because the data collection strategy was developed for an overall program evaluation, and not the study described in this paper.

One-way this unevenness was manifested was that more file data was available than interview data. The interview data was gathered in the first six months of that the facility operated, but the file data described the first two years of the program's operation. The interview data was from youth who entered the residence during the transition from house parent to the hybrid model. Therefore, these were youth experienced caregiving from both models. This dual exposure could have affected outcomes. If we had youth who had only one model exclusively we might have found more distinct differences on the outcome variables. Therefore, the presentation of results should be looked at as descriptive and suggestive rather than as definitive. A clearer basis for judgment on what caregiver model provides for the best outcomes. However, the unique nature of the study site where both care giving models are available, partially off sets those limitations. This "experiment that occurred in nature" is not likely to occur often.

A further limitation is the definition of continuity utilized in the study. The definition relied on the amount of contact time between caretaker and youth, may simplify the concept. Continuity has a qualitative component that this study did not measure.

DISCUSSION

The primary purposes of this study were to examine if differences could be found in care giving continuity between the two models, and whether continuity had an affect on program outcomes. The child welfare literature suggests continuity of caregivers is not a trivial matter with youth in care given their experience with trauma, disruption, and loss. House parents provided more continuity, and were less likely to turnover, than were the child care workers. However, the type of caregiver did not have as much of an effect on the outcome measure as did the amount of continuity experienced from a caregiver. Youth could have received high levels of continuity from either of the care giving models. Higher levels of continuity were associated with a youth reporting fewer behavioral problems. The effect on behavioral problems was most apparent with internalizing problems. Less continuity meant more internalizing problems. Perhaps without significant contact with a caregiver the youth does not feel comfortable with expressing problems to care giving staff, and are thus more likely to internalize problems. Further research is needed to demonstrate the effect with larger samples in different settings, and to determine what effect differences continuity in has on other program outcomes for youth. Moving between cottages was not associated with a youth having more behavioral problems, but a move may have had some small negative effect on the acquisition of independent living skills. Moving within the residential facility does not appear to carry the same risk as placement change, perhaps because some semblance of continuity can be maintained in the facility. Youth still have with some of the same caregivers. A change of caretakers was also strongly associated with reporting more behavioral problems. However, since the turnover data are cross-sectional, we cannot say that these outcomes were a cause rather than an outcome of moving. It is possible that youth problems caused a worker to leave the cottage.

More continuity may mean that the worker had more time to develop the kind of relationship that would enable the caregiver to identify, understand, and address each youth's particular set of strengths and needs. A worker who has continual contact with a youth has more of an opportunity to respond in a timely manner to resident's needs, and is therefore more likely to be viewed as responsive by the youth.

This study provides data to suggest that continuity of care is an important variable to consider in residential care, and it may be more important than the type of caregiver model. Unfortunately it appears that economics and/or state labor laws may be more significant variables in choosing residential staffing patterns rather than the best evidence involved. More consideration needs to be given of the use of the house parent model, or for designing the child care worker's job to make it more continuous for children and youth. Program administrators should arrange schedules in a way that maximizes the opportunity for youth to establish continuous relationships with the same staff. Child care workers could be assigned to a single cottage or shift in order to assure more consistent care giving. Residential placement agencies also need to address the reasons for high staff turnover that reduces continuity that youth experience with staff. The literature also suggests that better pay and education might reduce turnover among child care workers.

REFERENCES

Achenback, T. M. (1991). *Manual for the Child Behavior Check List, 4/18 and 1991 Profile*. Burlington. VT: University of Vermont, Department of Psychology.

Anglin, J. P. (2002A). Creating an extrafamilial living environment: the overall task of a group home. *Child and Youth Services*, 24(1-2), 79-105.

Anglin, J. P. (2002B). Pain, normality, and the struggle for congruence: reinterpreting residential care for children and youth. *Child and Youth Services*, 24(1-2), 1-23.

Anglin, J. P. (2004). Creating "well functioning" residential care and defining its place in a system of care. *Child and Youth Care Forum*, 33(3), 175-192.

Armudsen, G., Pecora, P. Payne, & Szatkiewicz. (1999). *An intake profile of children in long-term care using the Child Behavior Check List*, Seattle, Washington: Casey Family Program.

Barth, R. P., Courtney, M., Berrick, J. D., & Albert, V. (1994). *From Child Abuse to Permanency Planning*. New York: Aldine de Gruyter.

Berrick, J. D. (1993). Group care for children in California: Trends in the 1990's. *Child and Youth Care Forum*, 22(1), 7-22.

Bettelheim, B. & Sanders, J. (1979). Millieu Therapy: The Orthongenic School Model. In J.DNoshpitz (Ed.). *Basic Handbook of Child Psychiatry: Vol. #3*. (pp. 216-230). New York: Basic Books.

Casey Family Program. (1998). *How are the children doing? Assessing Youth Outcomes in Foster Care*. Seattle, Washington: Casey Family Program.

Daly, D. L., Schmidt, M. D., & Spellman, D. F. (1998). The boys town residential treatment Center: treatment implementation and preliminary outcomes. *Child and Youth Care Forum*, 27(4), 267-79.

Devine, T. (2004). A study of ways a residential group care facility can foster resilience in adolescents who have experienced cumulative adversities. Unpublished Doctoral Dissertation. Santa Barbara, California: Fielding Graduate Institute.

Feist, J., Slowiak, C., & Colligan, R. (1985). Beyond good intentions: Applying scientific methods to the art of milieu therapy. *Residential Group Care and Treatment*, 3 (1), 13-32.

Fitzgerald, M. (1995). On-the-spot counseling with residential youth: Opportunities for therapeutic intervention. *Journal of Child and Youth Care, 4*, 9-17.

Glisson, C. & Hemmelgarn, A. (1998). The effects of organizational climate and interoganizational coordination on the quality and outcomes of children's service system. *Child Abuse and Neglect, 22(5), 401-421.*

Leichtman, M. (2006). Residential Treatment of children, and adolescents: Past, present and future. *American Journal of Orthopsychiatry, 76* (3), 1-18.

Little, M., Kohm, A., & Thompson, R. (2005). The impact of residential placement on child development: research and policy implications. *International Journal of Social Welfare, 14*, 200-209.

Moore, K., Moretti, M., & Holland, R. (1998). A new perspective on youth care programs: Using Attachment Theory to guide interventions for troubled youth. *Residential Treatment for Children and Youth, 15*(3), 1-24.

Moses, T. (2001). Attachment theory and residential treatment, A study of staff relationships. *American Journal of Orthopsychiatry, 70*(4), 1-25.

Newton, R., Litrownick, A. J., & Landsverk, J. A. (2000). Children and youth in foster care: disentangling the relationship between problem behaviors and the number of placements.*Child Abuse and Neglect, 24*(10), 1363-1373.

Pecora, P. & Gingerich, W. (1981). Worker tasks and knowledge utilization in group child care: First findings. *Child Welfare, 60*(4), 221-231.

Ross, A. (1983). Mitigating turnover of child care staff in group care facilities. *Child Welfare, 62 (1)*, 63-67.

Short, J. (1980). *Youth Corrections Group Homes in Utah: final report.* Salt Lake City, Utah: John Short and Associates.

Smith, D. K., Stormshak, E., Chamberlain, P., & Whaley, R. B. (2001). Placement disruption in treatment foster care. *Journal of Emotional and Behavioral Disorders, 9*(3), 200-205.

Smith, M., McKay, E., & Chakrabarti, M. (2004). What works for us–Boys' view of their experiences in a former D list school. *British Journal of Special Education, 31*(2), 89-94.

Szajnberg, N. (1985). Staff countertransference in the therapeutic environment: Creating an average expectable environment. *British Journal of Medical Psychology, 58*, 331-336.

Terpstra, J. (1998). *"Residential Child Care": Sounds Clear Enough, Doesn't It?* Washington, D. C.: Department of Health and Human Services Children's Bureau.

U.S. General Accounting Office. (1994). *Residential care: some high-risk youth benefits, but more study needed.* Washington, D.C.: U.S. Government Printing Office.

Wahler, R. G. (1994). Child conduct problems: disorders in conduct or social continuity. *Journal of Child and Family Studies, 3*, 143-156.

Wilson, L. & Conroy, J. (1999). Satisfaction of children in out-of-home care. *Child Welfare, 78*(1), 53-69.

A Social-Emotional Assessment Method for Young Children in Foster and Residential Care: The Attachment-Based Narrative Story-Stem Technique

Timothy F. Page, PhD
Sherryl Scott Heller, PhD
Neil W. Boris, PhD

INTRODUCTION

Young children in foster and residential care who have experienced maltreatment typically face severe risks to their social and emotional development. The well-known developmental risks they face, and indeed the major reasons for which they are often referred for residential treatment, include severe behavior problems, poor peer relationships, deficits in emotion regulation, academic problems, and psychopathology (Kolko, 2002; Wolfe, 1999). In the eyes of many developmental scientists, extreme forms of insecure attachment are among the earliest and most significant of developmental risks prevalent in maltreated children (Carlson, Cicchetti, Barnett, & Braunwald,1989; Cicchetti & Barnett, 1991). Extreme insecure attachments in childhood have been associated with a wide range of later developmental problems in childhood and adulthood (Sroufe, 2005). Assessment of social and emotional developmental risk among maltreated children, especially those in foster and residential care, should therefore include information about the child's attachment history and characteristics of the child's attachment style.

Despite the fact that best practice standards mandate standardized and comprehensive assessments within 30 days of entering out-of-home care that include information about children's social-emotional development (American Academy of Pediatrics, Committee on Early Childhood, Adoption, and Dependent Care, 2000), a recent study found that many states do not have policies in place to accomplish this (Leslie, Hurlburt, Landsverk, Rolls, Wood, & Kelleher, 2003). Even where assessment protocols are in place, many problems exist with common data collection methods, especially for young children. Psychiatric assessment, for example, typically involves the use of the American Psychiatric Association's *Diagnostic and Statistical Manual of Mental Disorders (DSM)*. Despite the widespread usage of the DSM for clinical diagnoses, evidence exists that the diagnostic categories of Conduct Disorder for children and adolescents and Post-Traumatic Stress disorder in young children, among the most common diagnoses of children in residential care, are often misapplied and/or provide little useful clinical information (see Cameron & Guterman, 2007 and Scheeringa, Zeanah, Drell, & Larrieu,1995, respectively).

Most developmentally-based assessments of young children typically rely on informants who know the children well. While these data can be extremely useful, the reliance on informants introduces potential sources of bias, especially perhaps for parents motivated by a desire for reunification. At the same time, it is very difficult to assess young children's own perceptions of their caregiving histories and social-emotional functioning directly because of their relatively limited capacities for self-reflection and verbal communication. Clinical assessments of preschool and early school-age children have traditionally attempted to gather information directly from children's perspectives with projective and semi-projective methods, usually involving play or other creative activity, to infer and interpret children's experience from their creative expression. Limitations in terms of standardization and empirical validation among these methods, however, have long been problems that have constrained their broad acceptance among research scientists.

The relative absence of reliable and valid assessment measures for young children, from their own perspectives, entering residential care is a significant problem. Children under the age of 6 are the largest group of children entering foster care systems, and they stay in child welfare systems the longest (Vig, Chinitz, & Shulman, 2005).

A recent analysis of 981 children, ages 2 and above (mean age = 8.4 years), from the National Survey of Child and Adolescent Well-Being (NSCAW), a representative national sample of children in the child welfare system, showed that many children who enter out-of-home care for the first time are placed in intensive or restrictive residential placements, the result, in part, of serious behavioral and mental health problems. The typical placement, however, did not provide adequate treatment for the range of needs and problems the children faced (James, Leslie, Hurlburt, Slymen, Landsverk, Davis, Mathiesen, & Zhang, 2006).

There is, therefore, a compelling need for evidence-based, psychosocial assessments for young children entering out-of-home care that are sensitive to their developmental needs. Without such assessments, there will be limited understanding of children's needs, and thus the development of better evidence-based treatments is likely to remain very problematic.

This paper describes one evidence-based assessment protocol for young children, the Narrative Story-Stem Technique (NSST; Page, 2001). The NSST is used for children of approximately ages 4-9, a period for which very few standardized assessment measures from the child's point of view exist. The NSST was developed by attachment researchers who sought to learn more about children's perceptions of their caregiving environments. A case study of its application with a pair of fraternal twins with histories of severe maltreatment and foster placements will be presented.

ATTACHMENT AND ATTACHMENT BEHAVIOR

Attachment research over the past 30-plus years has demonstrated the central role in human development of the formation of attachment in infancy. According to Bowlby's original theory (1982), humans are born with a genetically inherited instinct to seek physical proximity with a known protective person in circumstances of distress. He referred to this instinct as "attachment behavior." The capacity to organize and activate attachment behavior becomes fully operational for most children sometime in the second half of the first year. Through accumulated experience with specific caregivers, the growing child learns about the predictability of available care and protection, and as a result develops an internalized sense of emotional security when his/her needs for care have been adequately met. The affectional bond of child to caregiver upon which this sense of security is based is referred to as the "attachment." Conversely, when children experience significantly inadequate care, they are likely to develop insecure attachments that reflect the nature of caregivers' inabilities to provide adequate care. Attachment security has been shown to predict children's personal and interpersonal capacities in several important developmental domains, including emotion regulation, self-image, some cognitive and social competencies, and, in extreme situations, some forms of psychopathology (Sroufe, 2005; vanIjindoorn & Sagi, 1999).

ATTACHMENT AND COGNITION

Bowlby proposed that accumulated memories of the ways in which caregivers respond to a child's activated attachment behavior become organized in cognitive structures which he called "internal working models" (1973, 1982), a term first used by the philosopher and cognitive psychologist Kenneth Craik. He chose this term because it reflects the mutability of these structures while at the same time communicating a sense of their relatively enduring nature. Internal working models are essentially internalized relationship qualities, the essential function of which is to predict the likely responses of others in situations where the growing child needs support or comfort. Evidence from attachment and social cognition research suggests that expectations of support and care in close relationships are predicted by secure attachments (Sroufe, 2005). In contrast, expectations and attributions of hostility in the intentions of others are associated with personal experience with hostile and/or unresponsive caregivers (Dodge, Pettit, & Bates, 1994).

THE NARRATIVE STORY-STEM COMPLETION TASK (NSST)

The Narrative Story-Stem Technique (NSST) is the generic term for an attachment-based method designed to assess young children's internal working models of attachment and other close relationships, particularly the qualities of children's organization of perceptions of caregiving relationships (Buchsbaum, Toth, Clyman, Cicchetti, & Emde, 1992; Page, 2001). Other names for this method, which reflect variations in the individual stories used in the protocol, are the Attachment Story Completion Task (Bretherton, Ridgeway, & Cassidy, 1990) and the MacArthur Story-Stem Battery (Emde, Wolf, & Oppenheim, 2003). A related version with a somewhat different administration protocol, the Manchester Child Attachment Story Task, has been developed by Green and associates (Green, Stanley, Smith, & Goldwyn, 2000).

The NSST consists of a protocol of simple, semi-structured story stems that the examiner introduces to the child using a set of family figures or dolls and simple play props. Each story stem is designed to provide a mildly stressful scenario that most children are familiar with (e.g., the parents go away for an overnight trip), and the child is asked to "show me and tell me what happens next." Children's narrative responses are coded for themes of interest. At present, several approaches to coding the NSST are used, though most of these code elements of narrative content, such as the qualities of parental caregiving, conflict, and the expression of attachment behavior toward parents, as well as overall structural characteristics of stories such as coherence and avoidance (Page,

2001). Research with the NSST over the past 20 years has shown that it can be coded reliably and that it has adequate test-retest reliability (Page, 2001). Its validity has been demonstrated in positive associations of it with measures of children's attachment as well as indices of psycho-social functioning (Page, 2001). Although most of the research with the NSST has been conducted with European-American children, it has also been studied with African-American children (Robinson & Mantz-Simmons, 2003), and with children in Israel and several countries in Europe (see Emde, Wolf, & Oppenheim, 2003).

Securely attached children tend to create narratives with the NSST that are characterized by logical and coherent story structure, with clear parental authority and nurture, expressions of attachment behavior, and positive resolutions (Emde, Wolf, & Oppenheim, 2003). Toth, Maughan, Todd Manly, Spagnola, and Cicchetti (2002) recently showed that children's representations of parents with the NSST were related to their parents' actual distress and, importantly, their improvement in parenting skills following a parenting intervention, as measured in pre- and post-tests. This important study provides further evidence that children's narrative creations reflect their perceptions of their immediate caregiving environments, and that these perceptions are mutable in relation to changes in those environments.

Applications of the NSST with Maltreated Children and Clinical Samples

Most of the early studies done with the NSST focused on establishing important, fundamental knowledge about how children can communicate in narrative form, and linkages between this narrative measure and other major developmental indices, including social behavior and attachment security. Since these early studies, the NSST has become increasingly used with clinical samples to better understand the developmental and mental health needs of children with psycho-social problems. A special issue of *Attachment and Human Development,* to be published in 2007, is devoted to several recent clinical applications.

More clinically focused studies have shown that the NSST can assess critical developmental and psycho-social issues, as perceived by children, including the reliability and authority of caregivers for consistent comfort, safety, and protection, children's pro-social and aggressive behavior, and the experience of intense fear, family conflict and instability (Buchsbaum, Toth, Clyman, Cicchetti, & Emde, 1992; Hodges, Steele, Hillman, Henderson, & Kaniuk, 2003; Toth, Cicchetti, MacFie, Maughan,

& VanMeenen, 2000). Several studies have shown that the NSST can be used to reliably discriminate between maltreated and non-maltreated children, and even distinguish narrative elements associated with specific types of maltreatment on the basis of characteristics such as portrayals of negative maternal and child representations, positive child representations, controlling behavior, the quality of the interaction with the examiner (Toth, Cicchetti, MacFie, & Emde, 1997), narrative and participant responses to story stems addressed at relief of distress (MacFie, Toth, Rogosch, Robinson, Emde, & Cicchetti, 1999), and core relational themes such as help-seeking, depictions of sadness or anger, and mutuality (Waldinger, Toth, & Gerber, 2001). In a related line of research, MacFie, Cicchetti, and Toth (2001) showed that sexually and physically abused pre-school-aged children created narratives with the NSST with more dissociative elements than a comparison group of non-maltreated children, and that these representations were found to increase over the course of one year. Assessment information such as this, from the child's point of view, is extremely useful in crafting interventions directed at children's most pressing needs. The following case examples illustrate these points, showing how the narrative responses to the NSST of two children can point the way to important directions for treatment.

CASE STUDIES OF TWO MALTREATED CHILDREN

The two children profiled here, Claire and Bobby, are Caucasian, fraternal twins, who were assessed separately with the NSST at the age of 8 as part of a larger follow-up study of children previously maltreated in infancy. (More detail about their histories is available in Hinshaw-Fusilier, Boris, & Zeanah, 1999, and Heller, Boris, Hinshaw-Fuselier, Page, Koren-Karie, & Miron, 2006.) Both were placed in foster care for the first time at the age of 18 months as a result of severe maltreatment, including physical and sexual abuse and neglect. Between the ages of 6 and 27 months the children experienced 11 changes of residence and custody that included placement in 5 different foster homes. The children were assessed by an infant mental health team at the ages of 19 and 36 months, and 8 years.

The NSST was delivered by the first author, who was entirely masked from any other sources of data or history about the children, as part of the 8-year assessment. Ten stories were administered in the protocol (see Table 1). The total time for administration was approximately 30 minutes for each child. The coding scheme for the stories consisted of the dimensions of:

- Family relationship qualities: Attachment behavior; empathic responding; caregiving; discipline; conflict; role-reversal
- Individual character attributes: Vulnerability; autonomy; competence
- Distortions of narrative/bizarre elements
- Narrative coherence
- Engagement in the story process

TABLE 1. List of Story Stems

1-Spilled Juice: The family is sitting at the table and little Jane/Robert reaches for some juice and spills the pitcher on the floor.[1]

2-Hurt Knee: The family is taking a walk in the park. Little Jane/Robert tries to climb a "high, high rock" and falls off it, crying, "I've hurt my knee, I'm bleeding!"[2]

3-Monster in the Bedroom: It's bedtime and the mother tells little Jane/Robert to go to bed. S/he goes into the bedroom and cries out, "There's something scary in my room! There's something scary in my room!"[2]

4-Departure: The mother and dad are going to go on a trip for three days, and say to the children, "See you in three days, Grandma will stay with you."[2]

5-Reunion: The mother and dad return from their trip.[1]

6-Headache: The mother and little Jane/Robert are sitting on the couch watching t.v. Mom says she has a headache and she turns the t.v. off, and asks little Jane/Robert for some quiet. The doorbell rings and it's little Jane's/Robert's friend who asks to come in and watch t.v. because there is "a really neat show on".[3]

7-Bathroom Shelf: Part I: The two children are playing in their toybox and the mother comes in and says she has to go to the neighbor's, and the children are not to touch anything on the bathroom shelf while she is away. The children resume playing in the toybox. Little Jane/Robert cries, "Ouch! I cut my finger, quick, get me a bandaid!" The older sibling replies, "But mom told us not to touch anything on the bathroom shelf." Jane/Robert replies, "But my finger is bleeding!" Part II: the mother returns.[3]

8-Three's a Crowd: The older child and friend are playing in the wagon. The younger child asks to join them. The friend replies, "If you let your brother/sister play, I won't be your friend any more."[3]

9-Broken Cup: The mom sits on the couch, crying. Jane/Robert comes in and the mom says, "I'm so sad because I just broke the cup that you gave me."

10-Ball Play: Jane/Robert is playing with her/his ball with her/his friend, Sally/Pete. Suddenly, Jane/Robert cries, "Ouch! That hurt my hand!" Experimenter asks: Why do you think Sally/Pete did that?[4]

---

[1] From the Attachment Story Completion Task (Bretherton, Ridgeway, & Cassidy, 1990).
[2] From the Attachment Story Completion Task (Bretherton, Ridgeway, & Cassidy, 1990), with revisions by Granot & Mayseless (2001).
[3] From the MacArthur Story-Stem Battery (Bretherton, Oppenheim, Buchsbaum, Emde and the MacArthur Narrative Group, 1990).
[4] From Warren, Emde, & Sroufe (2000).

Relevant Assessment Data at 19 Months

At the 19-month assessment Claire and Bobby were each diagnosed with Reactive Attachment Disorder (Claire had inhibited/withdrawn type, Bobby had indiscriminately social type)(Hinshaw-Fusilier, Boris, & Zeanah, 1999). They were also assessed in the Strange Situation Procedure (Ainsworth & Wittig, 1969) to have disorganized attachments. Additionally, Claire was observed to have Dissociative Disorder. Both children were assessed with cognitive developmental delays.

Relevant Assessment Data at 36 Months

By 36 months, some stabilization was observed in the children's lives. A maternal aunt and uncle received custody of them at age 25 months, and soon after this adopted them. Behavior problems, however, were evident at this assessment. Claire was observed to be controlling in her interactions with her adoptive mother. Bobby was observed to be self-endangering in laboratory assessments and during home visits. Both, however, were observed to use the adoptive mother as their primary attachment figure, a significant, positive development in light of their earlier histories.

Eight-Year Assessment

By the 8-year assessment, the children had been with their adoptive parents for approximately 5 years. At this time, however, the parents were undergoing a contentious divorce. Claire scored in the average range on cognitive screens. Bobby scored average in math and below average in verbal abilities. He also had been diagnosed with dyslexia and Attention Deficit Hyperactivity Disorder, for which he was receiving medication. Claire scored in the borderline range on the externalizing scale of the Child Behavior Checklist, and in the clinical range on the delinquent subscale. Bobby's CBCL scores were in the normative range.

NSST Responses

Each child's response to 3 of the 10 NSST stories is presented to illustrate several salient features of the stories they created. In these we see important experiential themes that would be very valuable to use as an organizing framework for clinical intervention. The stories presented are the Departure-Reunion sequence, two of the original stories created for the Attachment Story Completion Task, and the Ball Play story. The Departure-Reunion sequence was originally created by Bretherton and colleagues to portray a representational equivalent of the well-known Strange Situation Procedure, in which actual separations and reunions of child and caregiver are observed in a laboratory setting, from which attachment classifications are derived. In this story sequence, which in this protocol appeared as the 4th and 5th stories, the separation is presented as the parents going away for an over-night trip, followed by their return home. In their absence the grandmother stays with the children. This specific story sequence has been studied previously by Solomon, George, and DeJong (1995), who derived attachment classifications from it.

The Ball Play story was adapted from an original story by Warren, Emde, and Sroufe (2000) to provide a deliberately ambiguous social stimulus. In it, two children are playing, when suddenly one is injured. The subject child is asked to explain what happened. Previously maltreated children have been shown to be more likely to make hostile attributions of the motives of others in socially ambiguous circumstances (Dodge, Pettit, & Bates, 1994). This story, which was presented last in the protocol, was designed to attempt to assess children's attributional biases at the representational level.

Claire's Stories

Overall, Claire's NSST responses were quite different from the type of responses expected from children who experience stable and consistently responsive caregiving environments. As noted above, these children tend to produce narratives that are characterized by logic, coherence, and efficiency of expression, with consistent representations of care and positive authority, attachment behavior, and positive story resolutions. In contrast, Claire's stories were characterized by frequent and abrupt plot shifts with intense, intrusive, and frightening imagery. The father figure was repeatedly represented as selfish, incompetent, and infantile, though these representations were offset to some extent by some limited enactment of the father in authoritative roles. The mother was represented repeatedly in much more positive terms, in caregiving and authoritative roles, though not absolutely so. Children were depicted in several instances as deceitful, engaged in stealing and smoking, for example, and very vulnerable, including repeating depictions of death or threat of death. There were repeating representations of robbery by strangers, the most dangerous in the Reunion story, where a robber "almost kills" the little child. Following are the verbatim responses she made to the 3 stories (E refers to Examiner, S refers to Subject).

Departure Story (Story #4)

E: The mom and dad are going on a trip. The mom says, "Girls, your dad and I are going on a trip. See you tomorrow, Grandma will stay with you." Show me and tell me what happens now.

S: (moves parents to car) They get in the car, dad drives. Grandma goes to the park with them (moves Grandma and children to the grass). They both . . . have bloody noses 'cause they fell down. Now they go home. (S moves Grandmother and children off the grass, closer to her.) And Jane told her sister a secret, "Let's run away." (smiles)

And then they're packing up their stuff when Grandma's at the door, um, at the kitchen (moves Grandmother to other end of the table), and they sneak out the door (moves children away to far edge of table). And they sneak right here, to the store and they're stealing candy.

Then Grandma goes where they were inside the store. They had candy all over their face. Now they're sick. Now they go to the hospital 'cause each got a nail stuck in their throat. They all ate a candy nail (smiles).

E: There was a nail in the candy? They got it stuck in their throat? (S. nods) Wow.

S: They're at the hospital (moves children and Grandmother to side of table). The end.

Reunion Story (Story #5)

E: Well, let me show what happens next. You know what? It's the next day and the Grandma says, "Girls, your mom and dad are home from their trip." Show me and tell me what happens now.

S: They get out the car (moves mother and father toward grandma and children). "Grandma (unintell.), did anything happen?" (Parents ask Grandmother for a report.)

S: (Grandmother replies) "Yes, the children went to the hospital 'cause they got a nail stuck in their throat. They were punished 'cause they sneaked out the house and ran away to the store. And then they busted their nose at the park and they had to go home and take a nap." The end.

E: Um hmm, so that's what she said. She told them everything that happened, right?

S: (nods) Now the kids are punished. (S moves little sister and big sister to the side.) They lay there. And now Grandma's, and now the parents are dropping Grandma off at home (moves all to the car).
E: Um hmm, dropping her off. And did anybody else do anything after the mom and dad came home?
S: (distracted with putting figures into the car) I don't know (unintell.). (moves the car with all inside) Grandma's at home (removes the Grandmother) (moves car back) They're home. Somebody went in their house (removes all from car). And it was a robber, and almost killed Jane (moves little sister apart from others).
E: Almost killed Jane.
S: Now they called the cops. The cops came but they weren't there when they came (sets all back into car).They left (moves car slightly) and they're back home. And the cops were there (removes family from the car) and they arrested him . . . But he got away. They almost arrested him. And then they catched him.
E: Oh, and then they caught him, eh?
S: Yeah.

Ball Play (Story #10)

S: (Sally says) "I'm sorry. I'll never do it again. Now let's play."
E: Why did she do that?
S: She (Sally) did it on accident, cause when she threw it (ball), it hit her (little sister).
E: Oh, I see.
S: "Now let's play." (S. enacts them passing the ball to each other.) Now the sister comes out. (Big sister asks) "Can I play?" (Friend answers) "Yes, y'all . . . you can play too."
(Little sister says) "No, don't let her play. She was mean to me yesterday."
E: Who said that? (S. points to little sister) Little Jane did? (S. nods)
S: (Mother and father are moved closer and big sister says): "Mom, Dad she won't let me play." (Father says) "Then you can't play, Jane. You are punished for doing that. Go sit in the corner." (S. moves little sister to the corner.) And all them played. (Father says): "We're going to play too. Family ball. And she (little sister) can come back now. (S. moves little sister back with the family.) Let's play ball." (S. has family in a circle with ball in the middle.)

Then they lose the ball. (S. pushes the ball away.) (Big sister says) "I found the ball. It's over there. I'll go get it." (S. moves the big sister to the ball and brings the ball back.) She got it. But the ball has no air in it now. (Unclear who is speaking) "Okay let's go get some ice cream then." "I'm gonna put the ball there." (S. moves the family) They're at the table. (Sally asks) "Can I come in there and eat some?" "Yes you can." (Sally joins the family at the table.)

And then once they . . . these fall asleep. (S. lays big sister, little sister, and Sally down.) And then they (mother and father) go outside in the backyard. (S. moves the parents and lays them down.) And then they (big sister, little sister, and Sally) go in the backyard (positions all together now, lying down). And they watch the clouds.

Coding and Interpretation

Family Relationship Qualities

Claire represents caregivers, parents and grandmother, as present and often in charge, as when in Reunion the parents return and request a report on how things went in their absence, and in Ball Play when the older child seeks the parents' assistance in resolving her dispute with her sister, and the parents give reasonable consequences for misbehavior. However, their authoritative control and protection is clearly limited and at times inconsistent, as we see in the intrusive threat of the robber in Reunion and in the grandmother's inability to prevent the children's deceitful behavior and endangerment. Despite some inconsistencies in the presence of caregivers, Claire does appear to perceive caregivers as sources of authoritative stability, structure, and nurture. This is consistent with her later developmental assessments that showed growth in her capacity to form attachment to her adoptive mother.

In her Ball Play story, despite the father's suggestion that all the family engage in the play, the plan unfortunately fails because the ball loses its air. This image conveys a quality of sadness, even though the scene has the appearance of resolution with the serving of ice cream. The introduction of ice cream at the end of a story that previously featured conflict or troubled family interactions occurred in three other of Claire's stories, providing a sort of immediate and comforting device for situations that were actually very frightening or sad.

Individual Attributes

The deceit and stealing represented in her stories is consistent with the behavior problems identified by Claire's mother on the CBCL. Several images of intense vulnerability of the children, particularly those from the Departure and Reunion stories, are of concern. Similar images appear in several other stories that Claire told. The image at the end of the Ball Play story, of the children lying on the ground gazing at the clouds in the sky is a repetition of an image she created in an earlier story in the protocol, and suggests perhaps a sort of detachment, which would also be consistent with her history of dissociative disorder.

In the Ball Play story we see a benign attribution for the child's accident. This is potentially significant in that it suggests that she regards peer relationships as essentially benign, at least without an automatic assumption of hostility, and thus potentially mutually beneficial.

Distortions of Narrative/Bizarre Elements

The intrusive qualities of several images in Claire's story responses, such as in the Departure story, where candy nails get stuck in the children's throats after they deceive the grandmother and venture away from the house to steal candy, suggest an absence of integration of frightening experience. Morphologically, these intrusive images appear similar to post-traumatic stress symptoms, which of course would be consistent with her history of severe maltreatment. Images such as these have been shown to be important characteristics found disproportionally among maltreated children (Hodges & Steele, 2000).

Narrative Coherence

The majority of Claire's stories were characterized by degrees of narrative incoherence, including most poignantly the Departure and Reunion stories. In these stories, the structural quality of abrupt plot shifts was often combined with the intrusive and frightening images referred to above, though not always. The abrupt and frightening plot shifts that occur in the Reunion story suggest that Claire had difficulty making up her mind as to which direction the story resolution should go: first the robber was arrested, then got away, then was almost arrested, then caught. This story process suggests that she herself does not have a consistent expectation of safety and stability. Claire's Ball Play story, however, also contained incoherent elements, such as the abrupt plot shifts where the ball is lost, then found, then it has no air, then all go to eat ice cream, yet these had less frightening qualities. In another story (not presented here), the presented stem has to do with the mother's request of the child to keep the television off because she has a headache. Claire's story begins with the parent and child discussing the television volume, then abruptly shifts to a wedding scene in which the parents are getting married. One cannot help but wonder about the meaning of this story in the real-life context of her parents on-going divorce.

Engagement in the Story Process

Claire appeared to be very happy to engage in the narrative protocol, never once complaining, asking when it would be over, or appearing to refuse to participate. She was also never provocative with the examiner, but instead was very responsive to the expected structure of the protocol. She responded elaborately to all stories. Her affect, however, was often noticeably flat and incongruous with the narrative content she created, especially in the stories where one would expect intense affect, such as the Departure and Reunion sequence.

Summary

Several themes from Claire's story resolutions could be used as important foci for clinical treatment. These include indicators of intense and unintegrated fears, perceptions of intense vulnerability of children which are juxtaposed with impulses to act-out antisocially, inconsistency of caregivers, and sadness related to the absence of family cohesion. Based on her presentation during the protocol, and repeating story images of detachment, clinical intervention could also be focused on problems in Claire's recognition and expression of affect. She showed little expression of attachment behavior in her stories. There are also, however, several notable indicators of strengths that could also be used as important foci in clinical intervention for further development and growth, such as the ultimate benign presence and authority of caregivers, expectations of benign and mutually satisfying peer relationships, and her responsiveness and enjoyment in the examination protocol, this last of which suggests that she responded very positively to activities designed to focus on and understand her personal perceptions and experience.

Bobby's Stories

Bobby's stories were similar in one important respect to Claire's, in that he often also represented children in very vulnerable circumstances, particularly in repeating images of injury. These images, however, did not generally convey the same sort of intrusive and frightening quality that

Claire created. Throughout his stories, there is also a sense of interpersonal detachment, with exaggerated independence of children. His stories contrasted with Claire's in that they had, in general, more coherence in plot development and generally more positive resolutions.

Departure (Story #4)

S: (Parents say) "We're leaving. You all can't come. . . .Told you, you have to stay with Grandma. We're going out of town, to see your grandpa." Then those left, got in the car (S places mother and father in car). Daddy's driving, to the rain. . .

E: (Taking car off the table) Then what happens?

S: Then the grandma comes, "Who's hungry?" (holding little brother up to bigger brother, apparently to show little brother saying this) "Oh great, I don't like grandma . . . I don't like grandma's cooking." (S moves children to the corner of the table.) Then they run away to their room (unintell.), and go to sleep.

(Grandma says) "Ooh, guess they're not hungry." She went in the kitchen (moves Grandma), cooked some yummy chicken and they smelled it. Then they got up and (unintell.) (children apparently eat the food that Grandma cooked voraciously) ate 'em all up. Then they got tired, went back and slept. The end.

Reunion (Story #5)

E: Well, do you know what it looks like to me? It looks like it's the next day, and here's what happens now. The Grandma says, "Boys, your mom and dad are home from their trip."

S: (Children say) "Yay! Yay!" (holding children in the air, as though bouncing with happiness) "Yay, yay, yay, yay, yay!" (in a sing-song voice)

E: (moving the car back to the table) Show me and tell me what happens now.

S: (Children run to meet mother and father in the car) The kids run all the way outside, and they was driving to park (moves the car closer). They got out of the car (takes mother and father out of the car). Dad gots out of the car. I'm gonna put 'em on the table (S positions all together, has trouble standing them up). They can't stand up on the grass. (Children say) "Yay, mommy and daddy's home!" "Yay, I'm hugging my daddy!" "I'm hugging my mommy!" (enacts hugging) "Ooh, Ooh, Ooh." Then they went all to eat chicken (moves children to an imaginary table, makes gobbling noise). And the boys ate 'em all up. Then the boys go to sleep (lays the children down, then lays the parents down beside them. Lays the grandmother down with them.) And the Grandma, too. The end. And they all lived happily ever after.

Ball Play (Story #10)

S: Then he (Pete, the friend) kicked. Then he (little brother) kicked, until they were playing soccer. (S. enacts Pete and little brother kicking the ball to each other.) "Boow, Ohhh, . . .Wahh" (S. enacts little brother getting hurt. Pete and little brother walk away.)

E: How did he hurt his hand before?

S: They were all in (unintell.) (Unclear who is speaking, apparently a parent) "What you want?"
(Little brother and friend apparently say this to parents): "I hurt my... We hurt our hands." And they went to sleep, 'cause they had a cast on their hands. (S lies friend and little brother down together.)

E: They had a cast on their hands?

S: And then he goes, plays with the ball, basketball. (S. enacts the big brother bouncing the ball.) He plays basketball. And then, "Owww. I broke my leg." (Big brother apparently says this to parents.)
And then he went, he broke his leg, and got a cast. (S lies big brother down with little brother and friend.)
And then dad went, and played basketball. (S. enacts the father kicking the ball.)

E: What is he playing?

S: Kickball. And he broke his leg. (Father walks away.) And he laid down and got a cast. (S lies father down with others.)
Then the mom went to bounce the ball. Bonk Bonk (The ball hits the mom on the head.) "Ahhh, I got a headache. I broke" (S lies mother down with the others) . . . and now . . . and they all broke the . . . everything on their body. The end.

Coding and Interpretation

Family Relationship Qualities

In the Reunion story, which, as noted above, was originally designed as a representational proxy for the experience of separation from an attachment figure, upon which the Strange Situation Procedure is based, Bobby enacts very strong attachment behavior toward the returning parents, the strongest such enactment in his entire protocol. The nature of this response in this story is typical of children with secure attachments (Solomon, George, & DeJong, 1995). This enactment, however, stands in marked contrast to other representations of family relationships, such as those depicted in the Ball Play story. Here, the children appear to seek the care of the parents when they are injured, though this is not clear, and in subsequent representations the family appears chaotically disengaged. Each family member becomes injured and in need of casts. At the end of the story, after the mother is hurt, Bobby declares, ". . . and they all broke the . . . everything on their body," an image of family disintegration. In the three stories presented here, parents and grandmother are not represented as being particularly nurturing or authoritative. The grandmother, for example, in Departure, provides nurturance in the form of food once the parents depart, but the children figuratively thumb their noses at this and only eat later when they decide they are hungry and when the grandmother is apparently no longer present. This is generally typical of the rest of Bobby's stories, where parents are present though largely ineffective and detached. Interestingly, in the one story earlier in the protocol (not included here) where Bobby creates a fairly strong representation of the mother's authority, she scolds the younger child for being mean. He undoes this character strength, however, by having one of the children's friends declare he does not like the mother, which sends her crying to her room, and like a child, with no supper. He then repeats this scenario using the father. The enactment of parental authority followed by an undermining image or reversal of this is a repeating theme in Bobby's stories. This suggests that he perceives the presence and availability of effective caregivers as tenuous. He is nevertheless very capable of strongly expressing his need and affection for his caregivers.

Individual Attributes

The theme of injury presented in Ball Play appears in varying forms in three other of Bobby's stories, though these other enactments do not involve the entire family in one scene. The most notable of these occurs in the Hurt Knee story (not included here), in which the story stem presents injury to the younger child as a result of his attempt to climb a "high rock." The repetitions, and the detail, of Bobby's enactments of injury are potentially significant because of his real history of self-endangerment, first observed by the treatment team 5 years earlier, at 36 months. The question of Bobby's perception of the availability of consistent care and protection that is raised by these images, particularly considering the ambivalence and ambiguity that characterizes his representations of parents, would be an important focus for clinical services.

Distortions of Narrative/Bizarre Elements

In contrast to his sister's narratives, Bobby did not create the same sort of intrusive and frightening imagery. As noted above, however, he did create repeating images of debilitating injury, as exemplified in his Ball Play story. There were also some unexpected and peculiar images, such as the children in the Departure story complaining about the grandmother's cooking. In his Monster in the Bedroom story (not included here) he creates repeated images of the family figures as extremely frightened, though, individually, they alternate between being awake and frightened and sleeping. He creates these images of alternating states so quickly that the impression is that fear and sleep are linked in one process, in each individual. He also enacts some figures dragging others, who are sleeping, from room to room, presumably to protect them. As a whole, this story presents a very intriguing picture of consciousness and unconsciousness in the face of great fear.

Narrative Coherence

For the most part, Bobby's story resolutions were fairly coherent, in that plot elements were generally logically organized. The story resolutions themselves, however, were not uniformly positive, as seen in the Departure and Ball Play stories. Several of his stories, including the Departure and Reunion stories, end with the figures going to sleep. This representation, in an analysis by Solomon, George, and DeJong of these two stories, has been found to be associated with insecure-avoidant attachment (1995).

Engagement in the Story Process

Bobby was highly engaged in the story-telling protocol, never once appearing bored or reluctant to participate, and clearly expressed enjoyment in his interaction with the examiner.

Summary

There are several individual and relational themes presented in Bobby's narratives that would be potentially important foci for clinical intervention. There is a recurring sense of detachment and disengagement from other family members, characterizations of caregivers as ineffective, and a poignant sense of vulnerability of children. Similar to his sister Claire's narrative portrayals, one has the sense that children are endangered, though the form and intensity of this theme in their narratives differs. Bobby also appears to attempt to shut frightening experience out of conscious awareness, as seen in his frequent repetition of sleep as a story resolution.

There are also several noteworthy strengths he presents in his narratives that would be valuable in clinical intervention, most notably his capacity to express attachment needs. He also has very well-adapted interpersonal skills as seen in his responsiveness to the examiner in the story protocol.

IMPLICATIONS FOR PRACTICE IN FOSTER CARE AND RESIDENTIAL SETTINGS

Services for children in foster and residential care must reflect the developmental needs and challenges they face as a result of the inadequate care and maltreatment they have experienced. Developmental theory and recent research has shown that among their greatest needs is the stable presence of a committed, nurturing caregiver (Dozier & Lindhiem, 2006). This paper has shown how two fraternal twins with histories of extreme maltreatment and caregiver instability were able to communicate their perceptions of the uncertainty and instability of their caregiving environments through a narrative method. Details from their narratives provide important information for the direction of clinical interventions. While both created strong images of children's vulnerability and the absence or attenuation of consistent care, they did this in very different ways. The imagery that Claire created was much more suggestive of intrusive, frightening, and incoherent perceptions than Bobby's, though Bobby created more images of self-injury and inadequate responsiveness of caregivers. Through such similarities and differences, one can conceive how therapeutic intervention could be more individually tailored to reflect their differing perceptions and needs. Assessment such as that provided by the NSST, therefore, provides potentially rich data about the internal experience of children that would not otherwise be likely to be available from informant reports. As several other investigators have also pointed out, the representational format of the NSST has the additional advantage of providing the child an opportunity for the expression of painful emotional material that would not be available through a direct interview format (Buchsbaum, Toth, Clyman, Cicchetti, & Emde, 1992).

It may be that the NSST is capable of detecting, in particular, the presence of post-traumatic stress symptoms, though no specific research has yet been done in this area. Claire, who had a history of early dissociative disorder, displayed many frightening images that were presented in her stories with intrusive force that were suggestive of post-traumatic symptoms. Previous research has shown that dissociation among maltreated children can be assessed with the NSST (MacFie, Cicchetti, & Toth, 2001). Future research will be needed to examine more closely whether such narrative representations are in fact specifically reflective of post-traumatic stress symptoms, as their quality suggests. If the NSST is shown through future research to provide more diagnostic utility beyond the current evidence base of discriminant and convergent validity already evident, its importance as a clinical tool will only increase.

One caution that must be provided in the interpretation of children's narratives with the NSST is that our understanding of the extent to which discrete narrative representations reflect children's actual experience in and perceptions of social relationships is still in an early stage. Several studies have provided evidence that children's narratives contain much detail that is relevant to their psychological and social experience (Page, 2001). Much more remains to be learned, however, about the literal connections between children's narrative representations, their internal characteristics, and their social behavior.

Through a method like the NSST we are literally able to witness first-hand the concerns children have about their caregiving environments. The NSST allows clinicians and researchers to take the perspective of children, to learn about their experience from their points of view. The result is more sensitive and developmentally relevant assessment information and practice, and the expansion of the evidence-base of these activities. Clinicians working with young, maltreated children should thus contribute to these efforts by learning to use this method.

REFERENCES

Ainsworth, M. D. S. & Wittig, B. A. (1969). Attachment and exploratory behaviour of one year-olds in a strange situation. In B.A. Foss (Ed.), *Determinants of infant behaviour* (vol. 4, pp. 113-136). London: Methuen.

American Academy of Pediatrics, Committee on Early Childhood, Adoption, and Dependent Care. (2000). Developmental issues for young children in foster care. *Pediatrics, 106*(5), 1145-1150.

Bowlby, J. (1973). *Attachment and loss, Vol. II: Separation: Anxiety and anger.* New York: Basic Books.

Bowlby, J. (1982). *Attachment and loss, Vol. I: Attachment* (2nd ed.). New York: Basic Books.

Bretherton, I., Oppenheim, D., Buchsbaum, H., Emde, R., and the MacArthur Narrative Group. (1990). *The MacArthur story-stem battery.* Unpublished manual, University of Wisconsin-Madison.

Bretherton, I., Ridgeway, D., & Cassidy, J. (1990). Assessing the internal working models of the attachment relationship: An attachment story completion task for 3-year-olds. In M. T. Greenberg, D. Cicchetti, & E. M. Cummings (Eds.), *Attachment in the preschool years: Theory, research, and intervention* (pp. 273-308). Chicago: University of Chicago Press.

Buchsbaum, H. K., Toth, S. L., Clyman, R. B., Cicchetti, D., & Emde, R. N. (1992). The use of a narrative story stem technique with maltreated children: Implications for theory and practice. *Development and Psychopathology, 4,* 603-625.

Cameron, M. & Guterman, N. D. (2007). Diagnosing conduct problems of children and adolescents in residential treatment. *Child Youth Care Forum, 36,* 1-10.

Carlson, V., Cicchetti, D., Barnett, D., & Braunwald, K. (1989). Disorganized/disoriented attachment relationships in maltreated infants. *Developmental Psychology, 25,* 525-531.

Cicchetti, D. & Barnett, D. (1991). Toward the development of a scientific nosology of child maltreatment. In W. Grove & D. Cicchetti (Eds.), *Thinking clearly about psychology: Vol. 2, Personality and psychopathology* (pp. 346-377). Minneapolis: University of Minnesota Press.

Dodge, K. A., Pettit, G. S., & Bates, J. E. (1994). Effects of physical maltreatment on the development of peer relations. *Development and Psychopathology, 6,* 43-55.

Dozier, M. & Lindhiem, O. (2006). This is my child: Differences among foster parents in commitment to their young children. *Child Maltreatment, 11*(4), 338-345.

Emde, R. N., Wolf, D. P., & Oppenheim, D. (Eds.) (2003). *Revealing the Inner Worlds of Young Children: The MacArthur Story Stem Battery and Parent-Child Narratives.* New York: Oxford University Press.

Granot, D. & Mayseless, O. (2001). Attachment security and adjustment to school in middle childhood. *International Journal of Behavioural Development, 25*(6), 530-541.

Green, J., Stanley, C., Smith, V., & Goldwyn, R. (2000). A new method of evaluating attachment representations in young school-aged children: The Manchester Child Attachment Story Task. *Attachment and Human Development, 2*(1), 48-70.

Heller, S. S., Boris, N. W., Hinshaw-Fuselier, S., Page, T., Koren-Karie, N., & Miron, D. (2006). Reactive attachment disorder in maltreated twins follow-up: From 18 months to 8 years. *Attachment & Human Development, 8*(1), 63-86.

Hinshaw-Fusilier, S. S., Boris, N. W., & Zeanah, C. H. (1999). Reactive Attachment Disorder in maltreated twins. *Infant Mental Health Journal, 20,* 42-59.

Hodges, J. & Steele, M. (2000). Effects of abuse on attachment representations: Narrative assessments of abused children. *Journal of Child Psychotherapy, 26*(3), 433-455.

Hodges, J., Steele, M., Hillman, S., Henderson, K., & Kaniuk, J. (2003). Changes in attachment representations over the first year of adoptive placement: Narratives of maltreated children. *Clinical Child Psychology and Psychiatry, 8*(3), 347-363.

James, S., Leslie, L. K., Hurlburt, M. S., Slymen, D. J., Landsverk, J., Davis, I., Mathiesen, S. G., & Zhang, J. (2006). Children in out-of-home care: Entry into intensive or restrictive mental health and residential care placements. *Journal of Emotional and Behavioral Disorders, 14*(4), 196-208.

Kolko, D. J. (2002). Child physical abuse. In J. E. B. Myers, L. Berliner, J. Briere, C. T. Hendrix, C. Jenny, & T. A. Reid (Eds.), *The APSAC handbook on child maltreatment* (2nd ed.). pp. 21-54. Thousand Oaks, CA: Sage Publications.

Leslie, L. K., Hurlburt, M. S., Landsverk, J., Rolls, J. A., Wood, P. A., & Kelleher, K. J. (2003). Comprehensive assessments for children entering foster care: A national perspective, *Pedatrics, 112*, 134-141.

MacFie, J. A., Cicchetti, D., & Toth, S. L. (2001). The development of dissociation in maltreated preschooler-aged children. *Development and Psychopathology, 13*, 233-254.

MacFie, J., Toth, S. L., Rogosch, F. A., Robinson, J., Emde, R. N., & Cicchetti, D. (1999). Effect of maltreatment on preschoolers' narrative representations of responses to relieve distress and of role reversal. *Developmental Psychopathology, 35*(2), 460-465.

Page, T. (2001). The social meaning of children's narratives: A review of the attachment-based narrative story stem technique. *Child and Adolescent Social Work Journal, 3*, 171-187.

Robinson, J. & Mantz-Simmons, L. (2003). The MacArthur Narrative Coding System: One approach to highlighting affective meaning making in the MacArthur Story-Stem Battery. In R. N. Emde, D. P. Wolf, & D. Oppenheim, (Eds.). *Revealing the Inner Worlds of Young Children: The MacArthur Story Stem Battery and Parent-Child Narratives* (p. 81-91). New York: Oxford University Press.

Scheeringa, M., Zeanah, C. H., Drell, M., & Larrieu, J. (1995). Two approaches to the diagnosis of post-traumatic stress disorder in infancy and early childhood. *Journal of the American Academy of Child and Adolescent Psychiatry, 34*, 191-200.

Solomon, J., George, C., & DeJong, A. (1995). Children classified as controlling at age six: Evidence of disorganized representational strategies and aggression at home and school. *Development and Psychopathology, 7*, 447-463.

Sroufe, L. A. (2005). Attachment and development: A prospective, longitudinal study from birth to adulthood. *Attachment & Human Development, 7*(4), 349-367.

Toth, S. L., Cicchetti, D., MacFie, J., & Emde, R. N. (1997). Representations of self and other in the narratives of neglected, physically abused, and sexually abused pre-schoolers. *Development and Psychopathology, 9*, 781-796.

Toth, S. L., Cicchetti, D., MacFie, J., Maughan, A., & VanMeenan, K. (2000). Narrative representations of caregivers and self in maltreated pre-schoolers. *Attachment & Human Development, 2*(3), 271-305.

Toth, S. L., Maughan, A., Todd Manly, J., Spagnola, M., & Cicchetti, D. (2002). The relative efficacy of two interventions in altering maltreated preschool children's representational models: Implications for attachment theory. *Development and Psychopathology, 14*, 877-908.

vanIJzendoorn, M. H. & Sagi, A. (1999). Cross-cultural patterns of attachment: Universal and contextual dimensions. In J. Cassidy & P. Shaver (Eds.), *Handbook of attachment: Theory, research, and clinical applications* (pp. 713-734). New York: Guilford Press.

Vig, S., Chinitz, S., & Shulman, L. (2005). Young children in foster care: Multiple vulnerabilities and complex service needs. *Infants and Young Children, 18*(2), 147-160.

Waldinger, R. J., Toth, S. L., & Gerber, A. (2001). Maltreatment and internal representations of relationships: Core relationship themes in the narratives of abused and neglected preschoolers. *Social Development, 10*(1), 41-58.

Warren, S. L., Emde, R. N., & Sroufe, L. A. (2000). Internal representations: Predicting anxiety from children's play narratives. *Journal of the American Academy of Child and Adolescent Psychiatry, 39*(1), 100-107.

Wolfe, D. (1999). *Child abuse: Implications for child development and Psychopathology* (2nd ed.). Thousand Oaks, CA: Sage Publications.

Constructing an Integrated and Evidenced-Based Model for Residential Services

Jed Metzger, PhD

INTRODUCTION

Residential treatment for at risk youth placed due to emotional and behavioral health issues is a service facing significant challenges (Alliance for Children and Families, 2006; Pfeifer, 1996; Friman, Osgood, Smith, Shanahan, Thompson, Lazelere, & Daly, 1996). Challenges for residential services in this post-modern era are many and have been well described in recent literature. Most pressing challenges include; the high cost of care, often two to three hundred dollars per day of care (Lyons, Terry, Martinovich, Peterson, & Brouska, 2004), a reported inability to engage the whole family in the work (Skarich, 2006; Bullard, 2006; Carlson & Gabriel, 2001), a general lack of capacity to appreciate and appropriately meet the cultural needs of a population over-represented by youth and families of color (Capizzano, Adams, & Ost, 2006; Friesen, Kruzich, Longley, & Williams-Murphy, 2002), important questions of effectiveness of the service as a whole (Lyons, Terry, Martinovich, Peterson & Brouska, 2004; Shapiro, 2002; Reddy & Pfeiffer, 1997; Pfeifer, 1996), a paucity of evidenced-based approaches employed at residential centers (Burns, Rast, Peterson, Walker, & Bosworth, 2006; Yohalem & Wilson-Ahlstrom, 2007; Frensch & Cameron, 2002) and the lack of true integration of services (Lietz, 2004; Dennis, Dawud-Noursi, Muck, & McDermeit, 2002).

This descriptive, qualitative analysis describes the assessment and change process that a mid-sized multi-service residential center went through to address the above cited challenges and create an integrated, evidenced-based service delivery system. By engaging in a process that used assessment to guide the change effort, a focus on quality in the change process was facilitated (Wilson-Ahlstrom, Yohalem, & Pittman, 2007; Cohen & Austin, 2001). The assessment data was used to create a step-wise process to ensure systematic improvement.

THE AGENCY

The agency is a mid-sized child welfare organization that serves nearly 2,000 individuals a year in total and has 160 residential beds spread across campus, group home and supervised apartment program levels of care. The agency has a proud sixty-five year history of service and has numerous regulating bodies and is accredited by the Joint Commission of Accreditation (JCAHO). The agency has numerous long-term employees and maintains a strong record of developing staff through promotion and training. The residential programs serve male and female youth ages 11 to 21 who are placed by the Family Court/Department of Social Services system, the Office of Mental Health system, the Substance Abuse Treatment system. For the youth placed on the residential campus, there is a state licensed, 853 school. 853 Schools are not-for-profit schools that provide educational and related services to children suffering from handicapping conditions. The organization has a hierarchal organizational structure (Payne, 2000), so that the agency is organized top-down with senior administration divided between a programming side and facilities side. In the programming organizational chart there is a vertical line of reporting for each residential unit. In addition, all services have a vertical line of command based on discipline (social work, child care staff, nursing, education, and recreation); the consultant psychiatric and psychological staff tend to be assigned to units with only minimal oversight. This type of organizational structure is not uncommon and does seem to produce at least modest success when well administered (Payne, 2000). At the same time, prior to the reorganization, what can be described as squabbling between units and disciplines was also a common occurrence (Payne, 2000). Further complicating the picture was the fact that despite weekly clinical managers meetings, new initiatives were often not integrated into the whole. As a result, individual programs and/or disciplines would add or change programming approaches with little thought to the impact of these changes on the overall treatment intervention. While the agency was proud of its service delivery, historically well regarded by funders and accrediting bodies, the concerns and changes pressing upon residential treatment centers were increasing (Frensch & Cameron, 2002). The resignation and retirement of the senior leadership on the campus in the summer of 2006 provided an opportunity to reconceptualize and reconfigure the service delivery system.

Faced with a leadership void, growing concern over the lack of program and discipline integration and increasing pressure to provide evidenced-based care, the agency committed to a major system redesign. Central to the redesign was the idea that all change needed to be driven by assessment data (Wilson-Ahlstrom, Yohalem, & Pittman, 2007; Burns, Rast, Peterson, Walker, & Bosworth, 2006). Senior administration promoted the then leader of the group home and community residential programs to the new position of Residential Director. This individual has a long (27 years) history with the agency but was also known as a charismatic and creative leader who had long advocated for greater integration of agency services. Of particular concern was the issue of transition. Assessment of outcome data showed that youth were often successful while in care: They achieved measurable objectives on their individualized treatment plans, demonstrated school success behaviorally and academically, were compliant with mental health and physical health treatment and family members reported success in post-discharge outcome satisfaction surveys of the treatment. At the same time, when assessment was made of transition data, the picture was less optimistic. Youth were struggling with transition both within the agency (e.g., to a lower level of care) and in transition to the community. Gains made in care were not being maintained. The concern with transition is not an isolated issue and reflects the larger issues with residential care (Yohalem & Wilson-Ahlstrom, 2007; Lyons, Terry, Martinovich, Peterson, & Brouska, 2004; Shapiro, 2002; Reddy & Pfeiffer, 1997; Pfeifer, 1996). With the assessment data in hand, the new residential director and senior administrators pulled together a team of senior mangers and consultants and charged them with a two step process to redesign the residential services. The redesign team was directed to create functional units that could support transition and to integrate the programming with a mandate to employ the strongest evidenced-based approaches across the service. The team included the hiring of a former long-time clinical administrator as an acting consultant for this change process (author).

THE REDESIGN OF THE SERVICE

As noted, the prior design of the agency was largely based on a vertical management by of a level of care and by discipline. For instance, there was a director of campus who supervised all the social workers, and an assistant director of campus who supervised all the child care staff supervisors. This design had led to an often fractured approach to care. It was not uncommon for staff to actively engage in splitting type of behaviors when challenging issues arose in the work.

The agency had tried a small scale redesign in its group home program based on gender-specific programming (Hossfeld & Taormina, 1997; Miller, Trapani, Fejes-Mendoza, Eggleston, & Dwiggins, 1995), with impressive success (a massive decline in run-away behaviors and improved post-discharge success). The assessment made by the rede-sign team was that transition was perhaps the most critical area in need of quality improvement. Put together with the results from the gen-der-specific project in the group home, the agency was redesigned along these two principles while preserving the best parts of the vertical management system (Payne, 2000). A part of this approach was to use a practice where there was one overall administrator of any one unit that cut across disciples. This is a model that had been used in the group home program for a number of years with great success. To accomplish this aspect of the redesign, four assistant director positions were cre-ated. One for all the residential program beds for youth with mental health challenges (overwhelming male beds, 20 of 26 were male). One assistant for all the female programs, this consists of one cottage, three group homes (one of which is co-ed) and the largely female apartment program. One assistant for the male programs, which consist of two cot-tages and two group homes and one assistant for the brief and crisis resi-dences, which although have roughly equal male and female beds, are more focused on small brief treatment approaches and shorter lengths of stay (Hirshberg, Horgan, & Douglas, 1997).

Central to the redesign of the residential services was the belief that by linking the services based on the assessment of how a youth typically progresses through the agency, the gains made in any one area will be maintained (Frensch & Cameron, 2002; Dennis, Dawud-Noursi, Muck, & McDermeit, 2002). By linking the programs this way, greater consis-tency in interventions across the placement of any given client and fam-ily could be achieved (Lietz, 2004). In particular, the housing of linked programs under one administrator allowed for the program to be more responsive to family needs (Skarich, 2006; Cohen & Austin, 2001). Staff can be shared and longer term relationships with families devel-oped (Skarich, 2006; Shapiro, 2002). With a sharper focus on transition the new service directly attempts to address the concern raised by Shaprio (2002) of residential treatment being overly "context driven." Youth requiring the largest amounts of support do well in structured and controlled settings, but once those external reinforcers and controls are removed, the gains do not transition well to the community/family setting (Shapiro, Welker, & Pierce, 1999). As a way to increase the focus on transition, each new unit was restructured to create transition workers. The job of the transition worker was to link the youth as they moved both through the service and back into the community. The idea for a transition worker was taken from the State Office of Mental Health system which has employed this idea for the past four years with much success.

The redesign, while not without its growing pains also created staff synergy (Cohen & Austin, 2001). In order to capitalize on this synergy, each new unit began cross-disciplinary meetings to use the assessment of the challenges of transition to create greater opportunity to collaborate and provide holistic care (Payne, 2000). One fine example came from the recreational therapy workers assigned to each unit. The recreational therapy staff had come to experience themselves as the staff that took the kids and entertained them when the other staff wanted a break. The therapeutic recreation staff felt poorly integrated into the overall agency. The recreation staff rose to the occasion by requesting to do transition work with each youth so that youth had a positive community involvement experience. This intervention is driven by an individualized assessment and allowed the recreation therapists to link adventure-based learning to community connections (Neill & Richards, 1998). For one youth this may look like joining a local boxing gym, for another it may involve volunteering in an elderly care center, whatever the youth and family saw as important for transition (Skarich, 2006).

THE CREATION OF AN EVIDENCED-BASED, INTEGRATED MODEL OF CARE

The current landscape of residential services demands that in order for residential treatment to remain a viable service it must be integrated and apply evidenced-based models (Bullard, 2006; Frensch & Cameron, 2002). The group leading the redesign included leaders of all the major professional disciplines. The group was given the task to make assessment of the current programming and for each discipline to present a model of programming that could be both integrative and evidenced-based. Programming needed to be family driven (Skarich, 2006) and culturally responsive to the youth and families served by the agency (Capizzano, Adams, & Ost, 2006; Friesen, Kruzich, Longley, & Williams-Murphy, 2002). Overarching all of these important considerations was the issue of safety. The assessment was made that for the residential services to truly achieve the expected results, staff, youth and families needed to experience themselves as safe. Each discipline was charged with researching the various evidenced-based intervention models for their field and reporting back to the group so that a holistic approach could be planned. Each discipline was asked to bring forward models that were evidenced-based and reflective of the core needs of the youth for safety and successful transition.

In terms of the strongest evidenced based holistic approaches to residential programming, the *sanctuary model* (Bloom, 2005) has shown the greatest promise to rise to the level of an evidenced-based practice (California Evidenced-Based Clearinghouse for Child Welfare, retrieved 4/9/07 from www.cachildwelfareclearinghouse.org/). In searching for an evidenced-based model of residential care, the sanctuary model was the only full system approach so designated by the California Evidenced-Based Clearinghouse, which led to its adoption at the agency. From a practical point of view, the principles of the sanctuary model were fairly easily applied to each of the major disciplines at the agency (clinical staff, residential staff, recreational staff and teaching staff). The main tenets of safety, empowerment, and pro-social management of affect (Rivard, McCorkle, Duncan, Pasquale, Bloom, & Abramovitz, 2004) easily fit into the various approaches used but were now more focused and directed. Most importantly as increasing efforts are made to divert youth from residential placement and provide services in their homes (Lyons, Terry, Martinovich, Peterson, & Brouska, 2004), the youth that are placed in residential care are becoming more challenging (Shapiro, 2002). In particular, the number of youth with significant trauma history in their background demands that residential centers be able to assess and work with the effects of the trauma (Abramovitz & Bloom, 2003). The guiding sanctuary mantra of "it is not what is wrong with you? It is what happened to you?" (Abramovitz & Bloom, 2003) proved to be a conceptualization that all staff, regardless of discipline, could embrace. In an effort to integrate the concepts and to bring the whole staff together (Cohen & Austin, 2001); the training on the sanctuary model was done by unit with all staff present. Specifically, the training style was provided over a period of weeks at the scheduled treatment team meetings and was focused on application of the concepts. For instance, with regard to safety, the training began with didactic understanding of safety but then moved to all staff discussing how they create the various aspects of safety (physical, emotional, psychological, social and moral) in their programming, the threats to each aspect of safety and finally to apply those ideas to the specific youth and families in their care. Whole team training was provided by unit, with a focus on interactive discussion and application of concepts. This allowed for the overarching ideas of the sanctuary model, to be well integrated into the residential service. With the framework of sanctuary in place, the assessment team set out to have each of the four major disciplines identify an evidenced-based approach to be trained and integrated into the holistic milieu of the new residential service (Glisson & Schoenwald, 2005).

THE RESIDENTIAL STAFF

Central to the sanctuary work (Bloom, 2005) and good residential practice (Shapiro, 2002), it is important for the residential staff to both be viewed as, and to see themselves as providing clinical care for the youth. In their own language, "they are not babysitters." In order to more fully have the residential staff take on the mindset that they too, provide clinical work and to have the services they provide be coherent and integrated, it was critical that the staff be trained differently. Too often training for residential counselors in a residential program is largely focused on implementing agency policy with brief overviews of adolescent development and crisis de-escalation practices. Largely ignored have been the day to day therapeutic exchanges that define the job. Given the increasingly large numbers of youth with trauma in their backgrounds (Bloom, 2005), a model was sought that would address this issue. As the agency was proceeding by using assessment to drive change and wishing to be evidenced-based in all new applications (Burns, Rast, Peterson, Walker, & Bosworth, 2006), the decision was made to move forward with training the residential staff in *trauma-focused cognitive-behavioral therapy* (Swarbrick, 2004; Cohen, Deblinger, Mannarino & Steer, 2004; March, Amaya-Jackson, Murray, & Schulte, 1998). The Medical University of South Carolina (http://tfcbt.musc.edu) has a complete nine section on-line training curriculum covering subjects such as psychoeducation, stress management, and affect expression. Each unit has pre and post test evaluation, training and role play activity. The training was found to be easy to use, easy to administer and easy for the staff to apply. As the on-line curriculum training approach generates a progress report, it was easy to track staff progress through the curriculum. Additionally, the model related well to the work of the other disciplines, as it is empowerment and strength's driven (Cox, 2006) and reflects the need for innovative solutions to the current challenges faced by residential care providers (Alliance for Children and Families, 2006). Training for staff has always been seen as a priority in the agency. All trainings have strict attendance policies and a monthly report is generated which delineates who attended each individual training offered and for all staff who missed any given training what the rational for the absence was. The training attendance report is distributed to all management staff and reviewed by the agency president/CEO. Additionally, all participants in any given training fill out an anonymous training feedback form to track relevance of the training to the needs of the staff. To date, staff has reported strong support for this new type of training as it builds direct skills and is designed to be completed at their own pace. The trauma-focused cognitive-behavioral therapy approach has the added benefit of fitting well with the sanctuary model and this philosophical congruency led to the adoption of this model for the residential staff.

THE THERAPEUTIC RECREATION STAFF

The therapeutic recreation staff felt marginalized. Interpersonal exchanges with past administrators and agency drift had pushed the therapeutic recreation staff into a position where they were largely viewed as staff whose job was to "play kick-ball" and amuse youth, than as a critical and integrated part of the agency. The re-design team's assessment was that the underutilized therapeutic recreation staff was an ignored strength of the agency (Alliance for Children and Families, 2006). The therapeutic recreation staff had previously tried to integrate an experiential education program (Kolb, 1984) into the residential programming. When the redesign team looked at what experiential education is intended to bring to the residential setting, it was clear that a re-commitment to experiential education was essential to restore quality to this aspect of programming (Davidson-Methot, 2004). Rather than have the therapeutic recreation staff housed in the back of he school building and having the youth come to them, the therapeutic recreation staff would be attached to the residential units and given a regular role in the day to day operations. In their new position with the team, the therapeutic recreation staff trained the residential staff on the use of circle-ups and full-value contracts (Schoel, Prouty, & Radcliff, 1988). These experiential education techniques based on the theories of Kurt Lewin and Kurt Hahn, are empowerment based (Moote & Wodarski, 1997) and use action to create experience that is translated (processed) into learning with the youth (Luckner, Nadler, & Reldan, 1997).

Additionally, the applications of experiential education and adventure-based therapy have a long history of evidenced-based results with high risk youth and youth in residential settings (Neill & Richards, 1998; Schoel, Prouty, & Radcliff, 1988). Most importantly for this assessment-driven service redesign, the experiential education ideas and concepts fit into the overall strengths-based integrated model (Hirshberg, Horgan, & Douglass, 1997). The therapeutic recreation staff, once on the outside of the agency practice had been brought back into the center of the treatment. The effect of the circle-ups alone as a vehicle for creating experience that was safe (an underlying value of both experiential education and good residential programming) can not be understated. Now every individual at the residential setting- staff and client alike, were empowered to call a circle up and believe that what they had to say would be heard and valued. Empirical meta-analyses demonstrates that the gains made from these types of therapeutic recreational activities are maintained and integrated after the youth has transitioned back to the community, underscoring the essential nature of this service component (Neill & Richards, 1998). Finally the model, with the premium placed on safety was easily applied to the sanctuary model and was therefore adopted.

THE TEACHING STAFF

The agency operates an 853, state licensed school. By definition the youth in the school came to the setting with a variety of behavioral difficulties and past school failure. Prior to placement in the residential center, school experiences for the youth, were largely noteworthy for academic failure and behavioral consequence. While the school was seen as being largely successful compared to pre-placement standards, too many youth were leaving the school during the day to return to the cottages due to behavioral issues. Post-discharge satisfaction survey data found that parents were reporting that the youth struggled to maintain gains made in the residential school once they transitioned back to community school. In searching for an evidenced-based approach for the teaching environment, the redesign team quickly settled on the application of the *Positive Behavior Intervention and Support System* (Carr, Dunlap, Horner, Koegel, Turnbull, Sailor, Anderson, Albin, Kern-Koegel, & Fox, 2002). The school-wide system helps youth develop the skill set to manage the interpersonal dynamics in the school setting so that they may achieve academically (Beebe-Frankenberger, Gresham, Lane, & O'Shaunessy, 2003). The program is a large scale social learning model and as it is strengths-based, fits nicely with the trauma-focused cognitive-behavioral therapy of the residential staff and the experiential education of the therapeutic recreation staff. Each month the teaching staff would choose one aspect of the positive behavior matrix on which to focus. That aspect (e.g., respect) would be posted all over the school on banners, integrated into lessons, used in public announcements and communicated to the residential staff so that the cottage could integrate the idea as well. Behavioral incidents in the school showed a marked decline in the first three months of the project. This is consistent with the literature that positive behavior intervention and support system is an evidenced-based academic setting practice (Carr et al., 2002; Effective Practices, 2001). As with the other evidenced-based models chosen in this agency redesign, positive behavior intervention and support system values safety and democratic process, core elements in the sanctuary model. As the final model chosen in the redesign process, the fit with the guiding principles of sanctuary led to the smoother integration of this model.

THE CLINICAL STAFF

The clinical staff of the agency had long adopted a strengths-based approach to their work (Saleebey, 2002). The clinical staff had been training together on an every other week basis in this model for several years with mixed success. Assessment of the clinical practice across the agency showed a general lack of fidelity to the model, due to a lack of specificity in the application of the model. In addition, increasingly the main funders (Department of Social Services and the Office of Mental Health) were asking for evidenced-based clinical approaches. The local Department of Social services was moving towards the *child and family team* model that had been adopted by many social service agencies around the country (Kamradt, 2001). Central to this approach was the relational stance of "appreciative ally" that the worker takes in relation to the child and family (Madsen, 1999). The interest in this concept led the assessment group to Bill Madsen in Cambridge, MA. Madsen was brought in on two occasions to train the entire clinical team and to spend time with the clinical assessment group to design on-going trainings for the staff. This post-modern, evidenced-based approach was an excellent fit and addressed many of the assessed areas where growth was needed. The model is empowerment based (Solomon, 1976) as it directs the worker to join in a way and "ask questions in the service of the asking" that the child/family constructs their own reality (Madsen, 1999). The model demands greater cultural competency from the worker by explicitly placing the child and family in the position of power (Capizzano, Adams, & Ost, 2006; Friesen, Kruzich, Longley, & Williams-Murphy, 2002) and perhaps most importantly, is transitioned focused. As with any model, fidelity to the model is critical and the on-going training and supervisory monitoring for true application of the model is essential.

PUTTING IT ALL TOGETHER

With the discipline specific models in place, the hard, on-the-ground challenge of making the new service actually work together has become the on-going task. Central to the success of the redesign is open and transparent communication (Cohen & Cohen, 2000). It was important for leadership to communicate that the service was in a period of change and that, change can be stressful. The new director adopted a phrase, had it painted on the wall of his office and regularly used it to communicate a new culture. The phrase "Yes, and how can we make it happen?" became the mantra in the face of a wish to remain functioning as it had been (Cohen & Cohen, 2000). The new director developed a three and six month timeline for implementation of the plan. Once these were achieved a 12 month and a year two timeline were developed. While social service agencies are notorious for the number of meetings, it was critical to have regular communication meetings with the new director, the four assistant directors and the heads of each of the services to ensure that coordination and integration of the redesign was operationalized (Cohen & Austin, 2001). With regard to replicating this model of residential care, it would be critical to develop a strong communication structure and a culture that supported integration of disciplines.

The assessment process had also found that the agency needed to become more transition focused. To this end, transition became a major focus of the communication and practice of the service. It was critical for all staff to see residential as a transitional time in the life of a youth and family (Durrant, 1993). Being successful in residential care was only important as practice; the real challenge was to be successful back in the home and community. All staff needed to understand this concept at a deep level and use their specific interventions to build transitional success for the youth and family. As such, one message that was stressed to all managers was the need for the disciplines to integrate and communicate more. While being proud to being a part of the nursing or teaching team is important, the larger collective team and how that team works together is what drives success for the youth and families. This was a message that all managers were asked to convey directly to their staff.

Being transition focused was most clearly integrated by reconceptualizing the training program for the residential services. The agency moved away from large trainings given to primarily residential staff who trained as a cohort based on date of hire. While this had scheduling advantages, it meant that more seasoned staff had limited on-going training opportunities and that the trainings were generalized to the agency rather than specific to the team the staff actually was connected to. Training was redesigned to be delivered at the multi-disciplinary treatment team meetings. In addition to training the whole team at one time, this approach had the additional benefit of combining the didactic training content with application to the consumers of that particular team. The staff was asked to apply the learning to their clients, and this is a practice that creates deeper learning (Durrant, 1993). By training together the staff had an additional opportunity to work cross-discipline together as all disciplines who worked in any given unit trained together during the one time each week, when they were scheduled to be together. In order to accommodate the increased time demand on the training department, the agency doubled its full time training staff and increased the number of existing program staff who ran trainings, by one third. The fiscal commitment to the training department was added at the start of the second year of the redesign and this staff addition is viewed as reflecting the agency President/CEO's commitment to the agency redesign.

The agency historically has used a management by objective approach (Payne, 2000) and as a part of this approach, has administered a full staff survey every three years. The agency will administer the next survey early during the second year of the redesign with a special eye to the staff perception of the changes. Anecdotal reports form staff remain overwhelming positive, with the caveat that one program that used to receive a lot of the new director of residential services physical time, now gets less and misses the attention. The need to attend all staff being an important piece to keep in mind in all such restructuring/redesign approaches.

CONCLUSION

The process of redesigning the residential service is on-going. After one year, the redesign seems firmly in place, at the same time new challenges and opportunities arise regularly. It is important for practioners and directors working in residential services to see the residential landscape as in constant change here in the 21st century (Skarich, 2007; Hirshberg, Horgan, & Douglass, 1997). There is a place for residential treatment, but the service must address the current realities and needs (Bullard, 2006). For the service to be useful and relevant, it must be evidenced-based (Bruns, Rast, Peterson, Walker, & Bosworth, 2006; Cournoyer, 2004), family and youth driven (Skarich, 2007; Bullard, 2006), meet the cultural (Capizzano, Adams, & Ost, 2006; Friesen, Kruzich, Longley, & Williams-Murphy, 2002) and gender-specific needs of the clients (Hossfeld, & Taormina, 1997; Miller, Trapani, Fejes-Mendoza, Eggleston, & Dwiggins, 1995). Only in these conditions can the service provide the safety and transition oriented needs of the youth and families who are served by residential care.

REFERENCES

Abramovitz, R. & Bloom, S. (2003). "Creating sanctuary in residential treatment for youth: From the "well-ordered asylum" to a "living-learning environment." *Psychiatric Quarterly*, 74, 2, 119-135.

Alliance for Children and Families Magazine. (2006). "Old problems, new environments, innovative solutions," Spring, 6-11.

Beebe-Frankenberger, M., Gresham, F., Lane, K., & O'Shaughnessy, T. (2003). "Children placed at risk for learning and behavioral difficulties: Implementing a school-wide system of early identification and intervention." *Remedial and Special Education*, 24.

Bloom, S. (2005). "Creating sanctuary for kids: Helping children to heal from violence." *Therapeutic Community: The International Journal for Therapeutic and Supportive Organizations*, 26, 1, 57-63.

Bruns, E., Rast, J., Peterson, C., Walker, J., & Bosworth, J. (2006). " Spreadsheets service providers, and the statehouse: Using data and the wraparound process to reform systems for children and families." *American Journal of Community Psychology*, 38, 201-212.

Bullard, L. (2006). "Building bridges between service delivery providers, families, and youth." *Residential Group Care Quarterly*, 7, 1, 1-7.

California Evidence-Based Clearinghouse for Child Welfare. (2006). Retrieved 4/9/07 from www.cachildwelfareclearinghouse.org/

Capizzano, J., Adams, G., & Ost, J. (2006). *Caring for children of color: The child care patterns of White, Black and Hispanic children under 5. Occasional paper Number 72.* Washington, DC: Urban Institute.

Carlson, M. & Gabriel, R. (2001). "Patient satisfaction, use of services, and one-year outcomes in publicly funded substance abuse treatment." *Psychiatric Services,* 52, 1230-1236.

Carr, E., Dunlap, G., Horner, R., Koegel, R., Turnbull, A., Sailor, W., Anderson, J., Albin, R., Kern Koegel, L., & Fox, L. (2002). "Positive behavior support: Evolution of an applied science." *Journal of Positive Behavior Interventions,* 4, 1, 4-17.

Cohen, B. & Austin, M. (2001). "Transforming human services organizations Through empowerment of staff." In Tropman, J., Erlich, J., & Rothman, J. (eds) *Tactics and techniques of community intervention.* 4th edition, Itasca, IL: F.E. Peacock.

Cohen, R. & Cohen, J. (1999). *Chiseled in Sand: Perspectives on change in human service organizations.* Australia: Brooks/Cole.

Cohen, J., Deblinger, E., Mannarino, A., & Steer, R. (2004). "A multi-site, randomized controlled trial for sexually abused children with PTSD symptoms." *Journal of the American Academy of Child and Adolescent Psychiatry,* 43, 393-402.

Cournoyer, B. (2004). *The Evidence-Based Social Work Skills Book.* Boston: Pearson.

Cox, F. (2006). "Investigating the impact of strength-based assessment on youth with emotional or behavioral disorders." *Journal of Child and Family Studies,* 5, 287-301.

Davidson-Methot, D. (2004). "Calibrating the compass: Using quality improvement data for outcome evaluation, cost control, and creating quality organizational cultures." *Residential Treatment for Children and Youth,* 21, 3, 45-68.

Durrant, M. (1993). *Residential treatment: A cooperative, competency-based approach to therapy and program design.* NY: Norton

Effective practices. (2001). "Positive behavior intervention & support (PBIS) system." Missouri department of elementary and secondary education.

Frensch, K. & Cameron, G. (2002). "Treatment of choice or a last resort? A review of residential mental health placements for children and youth." *Child and Youth Care Forum,* 31, 5, 307-339.

Friesen, B., Kruzich, J., Longley, M., & Williams-Murphy, T. (2002). "Voices of African American families: Perspectives on residential treatment." *Social Work,* 47, 4, 461-470.

Friman, P., Osgood, D., Smith, G., Shanahan, D., Thompson, R., Larzelere, R., & Daly, D. (1996). "A longitudinal evaluation of prevalent negative beliefs about residential Placement for troubled adolescents." *Journal of Abnormal Child Psychology,* 24, 299-324.

Gilman, R. & Huebner, E. (2004). "The importance of client-satisfaction ratings in residential treatment outcome measurement: A response." *Residential Treatment for Children & Youth,* 21, 4, 7-17.

Glisson, C. & Schoenwald, S. (2005). "The ARC organizational and community intervention strategy for implementing evidence-based children's mental health treatments." *Mental Health Services Research,* 7, 4, 243-259.

Hirshberg, D., Horgan, A., & Douglass, D. (1997). "Acute residential treatment: Adapting our expertise to managed care." *Residential Treatment for Children and Youth,* 15, 2, 51-72.

Hossfeld, B. & Taormina, G. (1997). *Girls' circle facilitator manual.* Cotati, CA: Girls' Circle Association.

Larelere, R., Dinges, K., Schmidt, D., Spellman, D., Criste, T., & Connell, P. (2004). "Outcomes of residential treatment: A study of the adolescent clients of girls and boys town." *Child and Youth Care Forum*, 30, 3, 175-185.

Lietz, C. (2004). "Resiliency based social learning: A strengths based approach to residential treatment." *Residential Treatment for Children and Youth*, 22, 2, 21-36.

Luckner, J. & Nadler, R. (1997). *Processing the experience: strategies to enhance and generalize learning.* 2nd edition.

Lyons, J., Terry, P., Martinovich, Z., Peterson, J., & Bouska, B. (2004). "Outcome trajectories for adolescents in residential treatment; a statewide evaluation." *Journal of Child and Family Studies*, 10, 3, 333-345.

Kamradt, B. (2001). *Wraparound Milwaukee: Aiding youth with mental health needs.* Washington, DC: Office of Juvenile Justice and Delinquency Prevention.

Kolb, D. (1984). *Experiential learning: As the source of learning and development.* Englewood cliffs, NJ: Prentice Hall.

Madsen, W. (1999). *Collaborative therapy with multi-stressed families.* NY: Guilford.

March, J., Amaya-Jackson, L., Murray, M., & Schulte, A. (1998). "Cognitive-behavioral psychotherapy for children and adolescents with postraumatic stress disorder after a single incident stressor." *Journal of the American Academy of Child and Adolescent Psychiatry*, 37, 585-593.

Marsh, J. (2004). "Social work in a multicultural society." *Social Work*, 49, 1, 5-6.

Mattingly, M. & Thomas, D. (2004). "The promise of professionalism arrives in practice: progress on the North American certification project." *Journal of Child and Youth Care*, 19, 8-12.

Miller, D., Trapani, C., Fejes-Mendoza, K., Eggleston, C., & Dwiggins, D. (1995). "Adolescent female offender: Unique considerations." *Adolescence*, 30.

Moote, G. & Wodarski, J., (1997). "The acquisition of life skills through adventure-based activities and programs: A review of the literature." *Adolescence*, 32.

Neill, J. & Richards, G. (1998). "Does outdoor education really work? A summary of recent meta-analyses. *Australian Journal of Outdoor Education*, 3, 1,1-9.

Payne, M. (2000). *Teamwork in multiprofessional care.* Chicago, IL: Lyceum.

Pfeiffer, S. (1996). *Outcome Assessment in Residential Treatment.* Binghamton, NY: Hawthorn Press.

Reddy, L. & Pfeiffer, S. (1997). "Effectiveness of treatment foster care with children and adolescents: A review of outcome studies." *Journal of the American Academy of Child and Adolescent Psychiatry*, 36, 5, 581-588.

Rivard, J., McCorkle, D., Duncan, M., Pasquale, L., Bloom, S., & Abramovitz, R. (2004). "Implementing a trauma recovery framework for youths in residential treatment." *Child and Adolescent Social Work Journal*, 21, 5, 529-550.

Saleeby, D. (2002). *The strengths perspective in social work practice.* Boston: Allyn & Bacon.

Schoel, J., Prouty, D., & Radcliff, P. (1988). *Islands of Healing: A guide to adventure based counseling.* Hamilton, MA: Project Adventure Inc.

Shapiro, J., Welker, C., & Pierce, J. (1999). "An evaluation of residential treatment for youth with mental health and delinquency-related problems." *Residential Treatment for Children and Youth*, 17, 2, 33-47.

Shapiro, V. (2002). "Is long-term residential treatment effective for adolescents? A treatment outcome study." *Colgate University Journal of Sciences*, 155-179.

Skarich, M. (2007). "Redefining residential: Becoming family-driven." *American Association of Children's Residential Centers*. Retrieved from www.aacrc-dc.org March, 1, 2007.

Solomon, B. (1976). *Black empowerment: Social work in oppressed communities*. NY: Columbia.

Swarbrick, M. (2004). "A cognitive behavioral treatment program: Practical considerations." *American Journal of Psychiatric Rehabilitation*, 7, 193-199.

Trauma-focused cognitive-behavior therapy training course. Retrieved 12/28/06 from http://tfcbt.musc.edu

Wilson-Ahlstrom, A. & Yohalem, N. (2007). *Building quality improvement systems: Lessons from three emerging efforts in the youth-serving sector*. Washington, D.C.: The Forum for Youth Investment.

Yohalem, N. & Wilson-Ahlstrom, A. (2007). *Measuring youth program quality: A guide to assessment tools*. Washington, D.C.: The Forum for Youth Investment.

Meeting the Needs of GLB Youth in Residential Care Settings: A Framework for Assessing the Unique Needs of a Vulnerable Population

Rebecca G. Block, PhD, MSW
John D. Matthews, PhD, MSW

INTRODUCTION

Gay, lesbian and bisexual youth have different experiences and therefore different service needs than heterosexual youth. These divergent needs may be especially pronounced upon entry into the residential continuum of care. Based on differing needs, GLB youth are best served by residential care services that acknowledge their life experiences, and are sensitive to the challenges and risks they face. A key component to residential care is assessment, and assessment is therefore a primary focus and target for improvement of efficiency and efficacy of services to GLB youth.

The strengths perspective as set forth by Saleeby (2006) provides a framework to inform assessment that is relevant and responsive to the needs and experiences of GLB youth. Applying the strengths perspective informs the assessment process offers a variety of strategies and techniques for use in assessing GLB youth entering residential care. Through the lens of the strengths perspective, risk factors such as increased likelihood to use drugs, engage in unprotected sex or harm oneself are viewed as informative and not deviant. Experiences with managing stigma and making decisions about disclosure are key strengths as strategies for dealing with such challenges may provide invaluable support and information for coping with future challenges. The strengths perspective also provides insight into enhancing the empowerment environment to promote client centered and client driven treatment.

The manuscript provides recommendations for improvement of assessment with gay, lesbian and bisexual youth in residential care through a strengths perspective. A review of the literature focuses on both GLB youth as a population and residential care and treatment. Following this review of relevant literature are recommendations for assessment of GLB youth in residential care informed by the strengths perspective and a case example of these process and content strategies and techniques. Recognition of the unique assessment needs of GLB youth is the first step in making critical changes to residential care services in order to provide appropriate care for GLB youth.

LITERATURE REVIEW

Gay, Lesbian, and Bisexual (GLB) Youth

The difficulty in determining accurate parameters of the size of the gay male, lesbian, and bisexual (GLB) population in the US are well documented (Stacey & Biblarz, 2001). This is also true of the GLB youth population, who may be even harder to document than their adult counterparts. Difficulty aside, many researchers have attempted to explore the experiences of the GLB youth population, even without the ability to produce solid estimates of this population's parameters.

In Kinsey's (1948, 1953) seminal studies of human sexuality in men and women, it was concluded that approximately 10% of the population possesses a gay or lesbian sexual orientation. This estimate continues to be cited, referred to and generally accepted as the closest approximation available. Given that the American Community Study (2005) estimates the size of the youth (under 18) population in the United States to be approximately 73,131,688, there are potentially over seven million gay male and lesbian youth (10%) residing in the US, and countless others who identify as bisexual.

Until the 1990s, GLB youth remained largely invisible, even within the GLB community. Specifically, the existing body of research with this population has primarily used convenience samples of GLB youth utilizing community-based supportive services, such as GLB drop-in centers, GLB teen clubs, and HIV prevention education services. It is only in the last decade that GLB youth have begun to openly self-identify. However, even though this population is now more accessible than ever, there are new and complex reasons that explain the dearth of empirical evidence related to this vulnerable population. For example, Savin-Williams (2006), estimates that between 15 and 20 percent of adolescents have some degree of same-sex orientation, yet less than four percent embrace a gay or bisexual identity. To further complicate these issues, many of these youths do not link their sexuality to their identity, instead viewing the two independently. Without the link between sexuality and identity, it is markedly more difficult to conduct research with this population as many of these youth do not identify as gay, but variations that include queer, ambi-sexual, polysexual, two-spirit, bi-lesbian, tranny-fag, stem, stud, and boi. It is this variation that makes identification of, and engagement with, this population difficult.

Unique Adolescent Development Issues in GLB Youth

Adolescence is difficult phase of development for all youth. In general, this population has a variety of physical and emotional needs that are unmet. For example, approximately twenty percent are reported as having at least one serious health problem, and twenty-five percent are believed to be at high risk for school failure, delinquency, early and unprotected intercourse, or substance abuse (Ryan & Futterman, 1998, p. 3). The authors hypothesize that these problems may even be more pronounced in the GLB youth population due to the unique stressors, vulnerabilities, and health concerns of this vulnerable population.

First, the inherent difficulties in making the transition from youth to early adulthood are especially pronounced for gay male, lesbian, and bisexual (GLB) youth. For example, in addition to facing the expected obstacles of adolescence, GLB adolescents must master highly complex challenges and tasks, such as learning to identify and manage stigma. While any youth who experiences marginalization has to learn what it means to be an outsider and to manage stigma, GLB youth are generally the only group that is charged with making this transition without active support or modeling in the family. Further, because of the stigmatized nature of possessing a sexual minority idenitity, it is hypothesized that many youth develop the ability to 'cover' (Goffman, 1963), that is, they learn to compartmentalize their identity depending on their surroundings. With this in mind, it only stands to reason that GLB adolescents' major tasks related to identity development center on the consolidation of multiple identities, and the development of healthy coping mechanisms to deal with stressors associated with possessing a minority sexual orientation and identity. Ryan and Futterman (1998) refer to identity consolidation as the integration of one's sexual orientation within the context of their larger identity, and posit that this ability to consolidate disparate portions of one's identity depends on many factors, including individual maturity and experience, access to reliable information, availability of supportive adult role models, and sophistication or knowledge of peers.

The paramount goal of this life stage for GLB youth is to learn to manage stigma, which has serious social, behavioral, and health-related consequences. GLB youth most commonly experience "invisible stigma" (Goffman, 1963). This term refers to be largely invisible nature of sexual orientation. While outsiders may not be able to tell the person is GLB, the person is often aware that they are presenting themselves, their lives, and their circumstances in a manner that is less than truthful, and therefore often develop relationships with others that are rooted in a fear of being discovered, or found out (Ryan & Futterman, 1998). Finally, It is hypothesized that if one does not learn to effectively manage stigma, it can be internalized as self-hatred and low self-esteem. These attributes can then be acted out behaviorally, with an increase in high-risk behaviors, such as substance abuse, unprotected sex, as well as intensifying psychological distress and risk for suicide (Ryan & Futterman).

Common Disclosure Patterns Among GLB Youth

GLB youth typically begin the process of disclosing their "otherness" (hooks, 1992) in typical patterns. First, these youth must acknowledge these feeling to their self prior to disclosing to others. Once the process of self-identification is complete, youth typically disclose to gay or lesbian friends, close heterosexual friends, and close family members (siblings). The last two groups that individuals generally disclose their sexual identity to are parents and close friends at work (Herek, 1991). While the previously described disclosure patterns have remained valid over the past decade, it is important to note that these patterns are not the same for all individuals. For example, ethnic minority youth have lower levels of disclosure, especially to parents, extended family, and the broader ethnic minority community. (Ryan & Futterman, 1998, p. 18)

Common Mental and Physical Health Concerns

As has been documented previously in this paper, GLB experience unique stressors during adolescence. Some of the most common mental health concerns of this population include coming out to parents, coming out friends, relationships with family, sadness/depression, chronic stress, suicide and attempts, anxiety, interpersonal (romantic) relationships, personal growth, concerns about STIs, loneliness, alcohol and drug use (Ryan & Futterman, 1998, p. 28). Some of the common health concerns that are unique to this population include: HIV/STDs, reproductive and family planning services, trauma and sexual assault, eating disordered behavior in young gay men, substance abuse (Ryan & Futterman, pp. 42-43). While not true in all instances, it is often these social and mental health issues that are impetus for referral to residential care for GLB youth. Therefore, it is important to consider the different types of residential care available to youth in need, as well as the levels of treatment and restrictiveness of each of these levels to achieve an understanding of the options for residential care that exist for youth in care.

Youth in Residential Care Settings

Youth are referred to residential care for a variety of reasons. For example, a youth may be engaged in outpatient therapy with a mental health counselor, but experience a mental health crisis that necessitates a referral to a higher level of care. Further, a youth may also come to the attention of child welfare workers and be removed from the home due to abuse or neglect and be placed in the continuum of residential care, or may also be considered a runaway/throwaway. It is these two scenarios that are most common, and are the focus of the following section.

As of September 2005, there were approximately 513,000 children under the care of the public child welfare system in the US. More specifically, during FY2005, there were 311,000 entries into foster care, and 287,000 exits from care, with approximately 800,000 youth receiving some form of out of home during the year. (Trends in Foster Care and Adoption, 2006).

A demographic profile of youth in care during this time reveals the following trends. The average age of a youth in care is 10.6 years. Approximately 52% (n = 269,036) of youth in care were male, and 48% (n = 243,964) female. Without respect to issues of population size and disproportionality, the most common race/ethnicities included: Caucasian (41%, n = 208,537), Black (32%, n = 166,482), and Hispanic (18%, n = 93,996). The mean for length of time in care was 28.6 months and a range of less than one month to more than five years. Of the youth cared for in 2005, the most common placements for children include: non-relative foster care (46%, n = 236,775), relative foster placements (24%, n = 124,153), institutional care (10%, n = 51,210), and group home placements (8%, n = 43,440) (U.S. Department of Health and Human Services, 2006).

While the AFCRS report does not indicate the type of foster care (treatment vs. regular), the Foster Family-based Treatment Association [FFTA] estimates 11% of youth in out-of-home care are in treatment foster care (2004). Therefore, approximately 29% (n = 148,770) of youth in care in the United States resided in specialized, more restrictive care settings for a period of time during 2005. Finally, according to a national evaluation of the Comprehensive Mental Health Services Program for Children and their Families, there are five most prevalent diagnoses of youth in care. These diagnoses include: mood disorders and depression, oppositional defiance disorder, post-traumatic stress disorder, adjustment disorder, and conduct disorders (Austin, 2004).

Residential Care and Service Delivery for Youth

Residential care is defined in this paper as the provision of services to youth outside of the regular home setting. The most common type of residential care for youth in out of home care is traditional foster care, in which the focus is providing a substitute family structure for the youth in care. There is no explicit treatment component provided in the foster home; external services are secured to meet the social, emotional, and behavioral needs of these youth. However, some youth have care needs that cannot be met in this setting. Thus, they require specialized that generally center on more intensive service provision in more secure settings.

Types of Treatment-Based Residential Care for Youth

Once it is determined that a youth cannot be properly provided for in traditional foster care, there are more restrictive settings for providing services including the following: treatment foster care, group homes, residential treatment facilities, and inpatient psychiatric units. The causes of referrals to these specialized, treatment-based services generally include significant social, emotional, and behavioral issues.

Among treatment-based service options for youth in out-of-home care, treatment foster care is the least restrictive. Treatment foster care represents a model of care that provides youth with a combination of the elements of traditional foster care and residential treatment centers. It is through this individualized and intensive treatment approach that youth who would otherwise be placed in institutional settings are provided active and structured treatment in a home-like setting (FFTA, 2006).

Group homes are best viewed as small residential facilities where groups of youth reside in a small facility or single family home. While the group home represents a more restrictive and structured environment than treatment foster care, it is often viewed as a step down from care in a residential facility (Curtis et al., 2001).

Increasing in intensity of service provision, residential treatment facilities for youth represent an important component in the service delivery system for youth with extensive service needs. Programs provide for the educational, mental/behavioral health, and residential needs of youth in care in an institutional setting. Service provision in this setting represents one of the most costly methods of care, at a cost that is estimated to be 6-10 times higher than the costs of traditional foster care (Barth, 2002). According to the Substance Abuse and Mental Health Services Administration's [SAMHSA] National Mental Health Information Center, there were approximately 33,000 licensed residential treatment centers for emotionally disturbed children in the United States in 2000 (SAMHSA, 2002).

There are, however, many more centers, given the recent rapid increase in the number of private (unregulated) residential treatment programs in the US and abroad. For example, it is estimated that hundreds of these facilities have recently been established. The facilities and programs are often referred to, and marketed as therapeutic boarding schools, emotional growth academies, wilderness camps, and behavioral modification facilities (A Start, n.d.). As these are private facilities, they serve a different type of client than foster youth, with the primary target being those youth whose parents have the means to secure private treatment. It is estimated that these facilities serve approximately 10,000 to 14,000 youth in the US and produce revenues between 1 and 1.2 Billion dollars each year (A Start).

ASSESSING GLB YOUTH FROM A STRENGTHS PERSPECTIVE

The Role of Assessment in Treatment Planning and Placement

The concept of assessment is used in a variety of related fields including psychology, psychiatry, social work and counseling. Assessment is referred to as both a process and a tool in these fields for gathering information and determining an individual's current state. Some assessments are focused on one particular area of an individual's life or functioning, while others address multiple systems. Assessment conducted in response to a stated or suspected need for mental health treatment commonly addresses multiple dimensions including psychological, biological, social, emotional and cognitive functioning. The purpose of such an assessment is to gain understanding of client situations in order to identify a plan for intervention. In the process of assessment, a clinician applies knowledge from previous work and theory, in addition to judgment to explore, infer and define problems (Meyer, 1993).

Most assessments result in a report documenting the problems, symptoms and previous diagnoses held by the client. In addition to documenting the issues experienced by youth, the assessment process, which is most commonly used at intake, can also become a tool to develop treatment plans as a recursive activity useful for monitoring progress towards meeting established treatment plan goals. It is this use of assessment as a recurring activity throughout the treatment cycle that may serve as the foundation for increasing client's self-confidence and self-determination by providing a tool that can be used to chart progress, or exceptions to problem situations.

Strengths Assessment Framework for GLB Youth in Residential Care

While all youth could benefit from grounding the assessment process in the principles of the strengths perspective and guidelines for strengths assessment, gay, lesbian and bisexual (GLB) youth are likely to especially benefit from such an approach (VanWormer, Wells, & Boes, 2000). Looking to the literature on resilience, it is evidenced that protective factors have more impact when high levels of risk are present (Fraser & Richman, 1999). Similarly, it stands to reason that youth with greater numbers of risk factors present in their lives would experience greater benefit of a positive, progressive assessment process. Gay, lesbian and bisexual youth entering residential care are not only facing the same stigma, struggles and challenges that other youth entering care are facing, but they are additionally facing homophobia and heterosexism, whether internal or external, conscious or subconscious.

As discussed above, gay, lesbian and bisexual youth are at greater risk for substance use, suicide, to be survivors of violence and recipients of stigma than their counterparts. In addition, gay, lesbian and bisexual youth experience higher rates of ostracism and lower levels of support from family and other social supports including spiritual leaders, teachers and counselors. Greater levels of risk are based on the expressed or inferred identities of gay, lesbian and bisexual youth (Rivers & Carragher, 2003).

The strengths perspective provides a lens for assessment with gay, lesbian and bisexual youth entering care to inform both content and process, which is grounded in and consistent with social work ethics and values (VanWormer, Wells, & Boes, 2000). The strength perspective, as outlined by Saleeby (2006), is based on six principles, which include: (1) everyone has strengths; (2) painful experiences may be hurtful and may provide opportunity as well; (3) "assume that you do not know the upper limits of the capacity to grow and change . . . "; (4) collaboration is most effective in practice; (5) all environments have resources; and (6) social work is about caring and caretaking in context. In addition to the principles of the strengths perspective, guidelines for a strengths assessment were operationalized based on a social constructivism paradigm. These guidelines may be used as the interview schedule for assessment or integrated into the process and content of an existing assessment. The ten guidelines are as follows:

> (1) Document the story. (2) Support and validate the story. (3) Honor self-determination. (4) Give preeminence to the story. (5) Discover what is needed. (6) Move the assessment toward strengths. (7) Discover uniqueness. (8) Reach a mutual agreement on the assessment. (9) Avoid blame and blaming. (10) Assess; but do not get caught up in labels. (Cowger, Anderson & Snively, as cited in Saleeby 2006, p. 103)

The above principles and guidelines may guide the assessment process for gay, lesbian and bisexual youth entering residential treatment in several areas of process and in content. The strengths perspective in the process of assessment speaks to who is included in the initial intake assessment, how information is documented by clinicians and the perspective of assessment as a collaborative process for the benefit of the youth. Related to the content of assessment, the strengths perspective would indicate the reframing of some questions and the addition of others, as well as the integration of the guidelines for strengths assessment.

In looking at who is present in the initial assessment, there are often multiple adults present upon intake. In addition to the clinician completing the assessment, the youth's caseworker or family's caseworker (or both) may be in the room as well as one or more foster parents, biological parents and/or guardians. Allowing the youth to decide who remains in the room maximizes their strengths in multiple ways and on multiple levels. Being allowed to chose who hears their story can be empowering for youth, especially if they have had little choice historically about who knows what about them. The youth choosing one or more people to remain with them through the assessment demonstrates to them the social supports they already have.

Youth may be "out" to some people in their lives but not others; or they may not be out to anyone. Regardless of to whom they are already out, giving them control over who is in the room will create an environment to foster honestly. Youth being honest in their assessment about their sexuality, as well as behaviors and risk, will allow for services and service delivery that are more appropriate. Youth who are not out to the adults accompanying them and fear their finding out are likely to lie or leave out important information in the assessment to avoid being discovered or facing repercussions. Areas of information that youth feel compelled to cover may be related not only to sexual orientation, but also to risk behavior and strengths such as goals, aspirations and natural supports.

Documentation is an important part of the assessment process and an area that may raise questions for clinicians working with gay, lesbian and bisexual youth. Clinicians may not know how or where to document information about a youth's sexuality or sexual behavior, or if the information should even be documented at all. It is important for policies and procedures around documentation to be clear and consistent; wherein the same policies apply to gay, gay lesbian and bisexual youth as heterosexual youth. A strengths perspective indicates that all of the information documented be useful and relevant in supporting the client to mobilize their strengths. This provides grounds for judging what to document or how to document information provided in the assessment process, wherein clinicians may ask themselves–is this information useful and relevant in the mobilization of strengths for the client?

Both who is present in the intake assessment and the documentation of information shared in the assessment are related to and informed by the larger framework for the assessment. An assessment grounded in the strengths perspective is an empowering experience for the client, providing space for self-assessment, self-exploration and self-expression. Gay, lesbian and bisexual youth may be considered members of multiple stigmatized groups based on their sexual orientation and carrying a mental health diagnosis. Due to these and potentially other stigmatizing features, these youth may have been given little space to tell their story without judgment, to see themselves as capable and feel that they have the power to change their current situation. Entering into the assessment as a collaborative process of information sharing and information gathering to benefit the youth provides this space. It is from this stance that youth and clinician may begin a relationship that will best serve the youth throughout their treatment experience.

The content of the assessment may also be informed by a grounding in a strengths perspective, guiding the way in which questions are framed and by the addition of specific questions. There are several gender and sex related questions routinely included in an assessment, the first being whether a youth is male or female. This question is rarely asked, but one of two boxes is checked on a form based on the observation of the clinician. The first step in reframing this question is recognizing the difference between sex and gender, and identifying what information is being sought. Is the question one of biological sex at birth or current gender identity? Both of these questions are best asked as open-ended questions. Gender must be recognized as a continuum wherein individuals identify where on that continuum they fall. Sex is a function of biology and does not necessarily dictate gender identity.

Several questions in the assessment may be guided by the observed sex of the youth including questions about people important to them and sexual activity. Young women may be asked about boyfriends and young men about girlfriends. Questions about sexual activity may assume 'sex' is heterosexual intercourse. These are assumptions that cannot afford to be made; questions that may continue the marginalization of gay, lesbian and bisexual youth and promote the ongoing disempowerment they feel. Asking youth about significant others and with whom they are engaging in what sexual activities ceases to promote the heterocentric paradigm in a small, yet potentially significant way for gay, lesbian and bisexual youth entering residential care.

The importance of not asking leading or loaded questions is always present in assessment and especially so with gay, lesbian and bisexual youth related to behavior. Behaviors such as running away, using drugs or harming oneself are seen as inherently negative; looking at the meaning behind these behaviors and the strength in accessing coping skills, despite their lack of health or effectiveness, is informative and progressive to the assessment process. Gay, lesbian and bisexual youth may engage in behaviors that society may see as inappropriate such as enjoying looking at photographs of members of the same sex, interest or engagement in sexual activity with members of the same sex, or going to places known to be frequented by individuals who identify as gay, lesbian pr bisexual. These behaviors may traditionally be viewed as deviant or disruptive, but if the goal is mobilizing strengths, as reflected in the strengths perspective, these behaviors are self-expression not pathology.

In addition to framing existing questions in a strengths perspective, several questions might be added to the assessment. An important question to ask gay, lesbian and bisexual youth is to whom are they out, who supports them and what does support look like. Identifying natural supports is central in promoting strengths and healthy coping for all youth, and especially for gay, lesbian and bisexual youth as their social supports may be limited and may have changed based on disclosure of their sexual identity. Supports may include involvement in the gay or queer community and new friends and mentors who are gay, lesbian and bisexual. Youth may have become involved in social-recreational activities for gay, lesbian, bisexual and questioning youth, a queers and allies group at school or events at a queer community center. The social supports youth meet through community involvement may be new to youth, and may or may not know about other areas of the youth's life. At the same time, the some of the natural supports that a youth has depended upon for longer periods of time and who know about the youth's challenges and strengths in multiple spheres in his life may no longer be considered supports.

Asking youth how they have coped with challenges related to coming out or facing stigma or discrimination in the past is useful on multiple levels. Identifying past coping skills accessed allows youth to feel capable by seeing that they do have coping skills and have managed difficult times in the past. These skills may also be viewed as potential resources in managing current challenges including social, emotional, behavioral and mental health challenges. Past successes may serve as inspiration for future efforts to manage stigma, face challenges and make changes in their lives. This process is useful for all youth and paramount for gay, lesbian and bisexual youth as they have likely faced some kind of oppression in the past and are likely to continue to face oppression, even in the treatment facility. Most youth and workers in the residential care are heterosexual and have diverse experiences with gay, lesbian and bisexual youth. Treatment is set-up for heterosexual youth–rules about girls not having boyfriends and boys not having girlfriends, separation of youth based on biological sex regardless of gender identity.

While there are different perspectives on the benefit of identifying with a stigmatized group, most research indicates that identifying with a community or a group is more beneficial than not. Group identification provides support in combating stigma, access to individuals with similar experiences and a sense of belonging (Major et al., 2002). Gay, lesbian and bisexual youth would therefore be served by being asked about their group identification–do they identify with the queer or gay, lesbian and bisexual community? Are they involved in the community? How does community identity or the lack thereof serve them?

USING STRENGTHS-BASED ASSESSMENT WITH A GLB YOUTH: A CASE EXAMPLE

Joey is a Caucasian youth who grew up with his mother as his sole care-provider. Joey was placed in custody of the state at age thirteen after multiple calls to child protective services from teachers, neighbors and parents of friends. Joey's mother had multiple partners who often stayed over in the one-bedroom apartment that Joey and his mother shared. She was using multiple substances and just before Joey was removed form her custody, she and a boyfriend had begun making methamphetamines in the small residence. Joey's mother worked as a waitress at a neighborhood bar in the evenings and had held several different daytime jobs doing clerical work, and telemarketing, but did not remain in these positions long, as it was difficult for her to get to work on time and ready to work. Joey had learned to become highly independent, preparing his own meals, getting himself up for school and his mother for work and inviting himself to friends' houses when food supplies were limited in his house. Joey was not however able to protect himself or his mother from the violence perpetrated by some of her partners or her drug dealer. Joey managed to go relatively unnoticed by covering injuries, just passing in school and not confiding in anyone about his home life until he entered middle school. Until middle school, Joey was able to hide his home experiences, but when school and hiding injuries became more difficult, reports to child welfare began. As Joey grew, he felt not only more capable but obliged to protect his mother from violence. In his efforts to stand up for himself and his mother, the violence escalated and was brought to the attention of the neighbors. He sustained more severe injuries in the confrontation, which were more difficult to hide or explain away. Multiple reports to the child welfare system lead to an investigation and the eventual removal.

Joey was placed in a foster home with several other children ranging in age from four to fourteen. While his basic needs of food, clothing and shelter were consistently and reliably being met, his need to feel needed was not and Joey became very depressed. Anger and hurt led to self-harming behaviors, which brought Joey to the hospital for the first time. Over the next two years, Joey was hospitalized two more times, placed in three additional foster homes and one therapeutic foster home. After his second hospitalization, Joey was in a foster home where he seemed to be stabilizing. It was at this time that he finally felt safe expressing himself in small ways–hanging posters of young male actors he found attractive in his room, looking in the mirror and practicing how he will ask a boy to a school dance, telling another teen in the home about his perfect date with his latest crush. He was teased and harassed by the other children in the foster home, which brought out a violent response in Joey. Joey began beating up children if they gave him a hard time, and found that this allowed him to release his anger. Subsequently, Joey began punching and hitting other children in the home and at school without warning; he seemed explosive and unpredictable. This precipitated the third hospitalization and placement in therapeutic foster care. Joey is now fifteen years old, and after a violent altercation with his therapeutic foster parent that landed her in the hospital, he is entering residential treatment. Over the past three years, Joey has been seen by the school counselor, a clinician at the county mental health clinic off and on, and attended a group for children in foster care. Treatment has been focused on past trauma and current violent behaviors. Joey was diagnosed with depression, Social Anxiety Disorder and Post-Traumatic Stress Disorder, and prescribed a variety of anti-depressants and anti-anxiety medications over the years, taken with varied adherence.

Joey is accompanied to the intake assessment by his caseworker who has been working with him since he was removed from his mother's care and the mental health provider to whom he was assigned when he was placed in therapeutic foster care. The clinician asks to speak with Joey alone before beginning the assessment. At this time Joey is asked whom he would like included in the conversation. He chooses to have the newly assigned clinician involved and for the caseworker to wait in the waiting room. He later explains that his caseworker was very focused on his violent outbursts and could not hear anything else he was reporting. He did however, want more than one person in the room, as he felt safer that way.

Joey's assessment progressed following the ten guidelines set forth above. The assessment began with the clinician simply opening the floor for Joey to tell her about himself. Initially, Joey told the clinician what he thought she wanted to hear–about past violent outbursts, mediocre academic performance, the violence he saw at home and his mother's involvement with drugs and men. The clinician listened attentively, asked clarifying questions and encouraged Joey to keep talking, and he did. He told her about his childhood and the way which he thought he arrived where he was today. The clinician did not judge what Joey was saying and asked questions only to further the conversation, support Joey in his discovery and to see his own strengths.

Together, Joey and the clinician uncovered feelings that had gone unrecognized by Joey, his caregivers and his mental health providers. Joey expressed feeling different, angry and ostracized, and not knowing how to express these feelings. He had the opportunity to identify his coping skills, his ability to manage difficult situations and his resilience. The clinician used the language that Joey used in reflecting back what she was hearing from him; she asked for confirmation of accuracy and prompted him to share more as he felt comfortable.

After mentioning that he was curious about boys and wondered what it would be like to have sex with a boy, the clinician asked him about past experiences with boys, if he knew boys who had sex with other boys, if he knew adult men who had sex with men. She asked him what it meant to him that some boys have sex with boys and that he is curious about it. He reported not knowing any other boys who had the same thoughts and desires that he had, nor did he know any men who had sex with men. He stated that he knew that men who liked to be with men were gay and that there was a gay community, but lacked any further knowledge or information. He explained that he was given a hard time by other youth for talking about going on dates with boys and therefore felt like he should not tell anyone about these feelings. A distinct lack of social support emerged wherein Joey felt that he had no one in his corner.

While he may not have noticed, Joey was more honest and forthcoming with the clinician throughout the assessment. He discovered the coping skills that he was using, some of which had gotten him into trouble, such as becoming violent, and others that were more effective and healthy such as writing and drawing in a journal. While reticent in admitting it, Joey recognized that he had been through many challenging situations and still had hopes and dreams for the future, and wanted things in his life to be different.

The clinician allowed him to have power in the situation; she did not assume he worked from a heterosexual center and that his violent behaviors, or his fantasies about his future were deviant but meaning driven and illustrations of self-expression. The assessment clinician did not push Joey to interpret his behaviors further than he was ready and did not seek to label Joey based on his behaviors, and left the door open for such exploration to occur during his time in treatment. Using the components of a strengths-based assessment supported the creation and maintenance of an empowering environment, and allowed Joey to leave the assessment with his abilities and resourcefulness in mind as he entered residential care.

Upon completion of the conversation, the clinician wrote her assessment report including the information that was discussed. There was no question in her mind about what to document or how to document as the conversation Joey's narrative authored by Joey. The process of the assessment was focused on discovery of information that was relevant and useful for Joey to mobilize his strengths.

CONCLUSION

Identity development is a healthy and challenging part of youth development. This process becomes more challenging for youth in residential care, let alone youth in residential care who are gay, lesbian and bisexual. GLB youth residing in residential care are undergoing the processes of identity development and consolidation within environments that are rife with social disapproval, misconceptions, distorted stereotypes, and hostility (Ryan & Futterman, 1998, p. 22). Issues related to sexuality may be ignored by providers. The affects of experiences such as felt and enacted stigma, peer pressure, bullying and sexual debut may go unrecognized. Consideration may not be given to the ways in which these experiences are different, look different, impact different areas of life for LGB youth. Often, when sexual orientation is addressed, it can become an inappropriate focus of treatment wherein the treatment plan is written to address sexual orientation and related issues leaving presenting mental health and behavioral issues untreated. It only stands to reason that GLB youth are especially vulnerable when they require residential care. For example, GLB youth are sometimes subjected to reparative or conversion therapy (overt attempts to change one's sexual orientation) by those who are charged to care for them, even though these methods have been rebuked by professional organizations, such as the American Psychological Association and the National Association of Social Workers. A participant in a recent study (Smith, 1996) reported that two staff members in an institutional care setting told her that two thousand years ago, she would have been stoned to death [for being a lesbian]. Further, they quoted the Bible to her. While this is only one example of the maltreatment of GLB youth in care, this is clearly not an isolated incident. Therefore, professionals charged with providing for the needs of youth in out of home care need to develop a variety of strategies to support these youth applying theory and using techniques that are evidence-based, relevant and responsive. In order to serve GLB youth in residential care appropriately, staff must be properly trained through in-service staff trainings. Educating staff in addition to empowering youth may also occur through open forums for youth in care. And, as addressed in this article, assessment strategies that account for, and respect diversity among youth in care and the unique needs of lesbian, gay and bisexual youth must be implemented.

REFERENCES

A Start. (n.d.). *An alarming residential care phenomenon.* Retrieved on April 13, 2007, from http://astart.fmhi.usf.edu/AStartDocs/factsheet.pdf

Austin, L. (2004). Mental health needs of youth in foster care: Challenges and strategies. *The Connection, 20*(4), 6-13.

Barth, R. P. (2002). *Institutions vs. foster homes: The empirical base for the second century of debate.* Chapel Hill, NC: University of North Carolina.

Curtis, P. A., Alexander, G., & Lunghofer, L. A. (2001). A literature review comparing the outcomes of residential group care and therapeutic foster care. *Child & Adolescent Social Work Journal, 18*(5), 377-392.

Cowger, C. D., Anderson, K. M., & Snively, C. A. (2006). Assessing strengths: The political context of individual, family, and community empowerment. In D. Saleeby (Ed.), The Strengths Perspective in Social Work Practice (pp. 93-115). Pearson: Boston.

Foster Family-based Treatment Association [FFTA]. (2006). *What is treatment foster care?* Retrieved on April 13, 2007, from http://www.ffta.org/whatis.html

Fraser, M., & Richman, J. M. (1999). Risk, protection, and resilience: Toward a conceptual framework for social work practice. Social Work Research, *23*(3), 131-144.

Goffman, E. (1963). *Stigma: Notes on the Management of Spoiled Identity.* New York: Touchstone.

Herek, G. M. (1991). Stigma, prejudice, and violence against lesbians and gay men. In Gonsiorek, JC; Weinrich, JD (eds). *Homosexuality: Research implications for public policy.* Newbury Park, CA: Sage Publications.

hooks, b. (1992). *Black Looks: Race and representation.* Cambridge, MA: South End Press.

Hunt, M. (1974). *Sexual Behavior in the 1970's.* New York: Dell.

Kinsey, A., Pomeroy, W., & Martin, C. (1948). *Sexual behavior in the human male.* Philadelphia: W.B. Saunders.

Kinsey, A., Pomeroy, W., Martin, C., & Gebhard, P. (1953). *Sexual behavior in the human female.* Philadelphia: W.B. Saunders.

Major, B., Gramzow, R. H., McCoy, S. K., Levin, S., Schmader, T., & Sidanius, J. (2002). Personal discrimination: The role of group status and legitimizing ideology. *Journal of Personality and Social Psychology, 82*(3), 269-282.

Meyer, C. H. (1993). Assessment in Social Work Practice, New York: Columbia University Press.

Rivers, I., & Carragher, D. (2003). Social-developmental factors affecting lesbian and gay youth: A review of cross-national research findings. *Children and Society, 17,* 374-385.

Ryan, C.C., & Futterman, D. (1998). Lesbian and Gay Youth: Care and Counseling. Columbia University Press Publishers: New York.

Saleeby, D. (2006). Introduction: Power in the people. In Saleeby (Ed.), *The Strengths Perspective in Social Work Practice* (pp. 1-24). Pearson: Boston.

Savin-Williams, R. C. (2006). *The new gay teenager.* Boston, Ma: Harvard University Press.

Stacey, J., & Biblarz, T. J. (2001). How does the sexual orientation of parents matter? *American Sociological Review, 66,* 159-183.

Substance Abuse and Mental Health Services Administration [SAMHSA]. (2002). *National mental health statistics.* Retrieved on April 13, 2007, from http:// mentalhealth. samhsa.gov/publications/allpubs/SMA04-3938/chp18table5.asp

US Census Bureau. (2006). *American community study: 2005.* Retrieved on April 13, 2007, from www.census.gov

U.S. Department of Health and Human Services, Administration for Children and Families, Administration on Children, Youth and Families, Children's Bureau (2006). Trends in foster care and adoption, 2006. Retrieved April 16, 2007, from http://www.acf.hhs.gov/programs/cb/stats_research/afcars/trends.htm).

U.S. Department of Health and Human Services. (2006). The AFCARS report: Preliminary FY 2005 estimates as of September 2006. Retrieved April 16, 2007, from http://www.acf.hhs.gov/programs/cb/stats_research/afcars/tar/report13.htm).

Van Wormer, K., Wells, J., & Boes, M. (2000). Social Work With Lesbians, Gays, and Bisexuals: A Strengths Perspective. Needham Heights: Allyn and Bacon.

INDEX

A-B-C recording 38, 47–55, 57
academic settings 169–70
accreditation 162
action plans 19
activity schedules 109
adaptive behavior 46
adjustment disorder 182
administrators 83, 88, 96, 100, 107, 120, 134, 163–4, 168
Adult and Adolescent Parenting Inventory (AAPI) 5–6
adventure-based therapy 165, 168
AFCRS 182
alienation 71–2
alpha coefficients 126
Altschuler, D.M. 21
ambi-sexuality 179
American Community Study 178
American Psychiatric Association 137
American Psychological Association 192
analyses of variance (ANOVA) 91, 94–5
Andrews, D.A. 11
Anglin, J.P. 120–1
Annual Client Evaluation (ACE) 125, 129
Ansel-Casey Life Skills Assessment (ACLSA) 125, 129
antecedents 38–41, 43–52, 54, 108–10, 113
appreciative allies 170
Armstrong, T.L. 21
assessment
    behavior management 105–15
    client/staff satisfaction 61–76
    continuity of care 117–34
    evidence-based model 161–73
    functional 37–57
    GLB youth 177–93
    juvenile correction programs 11–28

social-emotional method 137–56
    staff competence 83–100
    substance abuse 1–8
Attachment Story Completion Task 140, 145
attachment theory 118, 120, 137, 139–41, 143, 145, 148, 150, 152–5
attachment-based narrative story-stem technique 137–56
attendance policies 167–8
attention 42
Attention Deficit Hyperactivity Disorder (ADHD) 105, 144
autism 42
automatic reinforcement 41–3, 50, 57
avoidance 42, 46, 140, 154

Ball Play Story 145, 147–9, 152–4
Barnum, R. 14
Barton, W.H. 11–28
behavior management 105–15, 120
behavioral interventions 85, 105–15
best practices 76, 137
bias 138, 145
Bible 192
biology 187–8
bisexual youth 177–93
bizarre elements 149, 154
blame 185
Block, R.G. 177–93
bois 179
bonding 139
Boris, N.W. 137–56
Bowlby, J. 139
Boys Town 87, 119
Bretherton, I. 145
burnout 61–6, 72, 74–6

California Evidenced-Based Clearinghouse 166